Finding Peace *by the* Sea

Finding Peace *by the* Sea

Inspiring Images and Quotes for Living Your Best Life

Harry L. Thomas, MSW

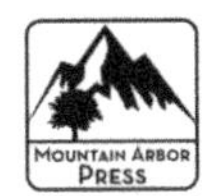

MOUNTAIN ARBOR
PRESS
Alpharetta, GA

ISBN: 978-1-6653-0292-0

Printed in the United States of America 1 2 0 5 2 3

This paper meets the requirements of ANSI/NISO Z39.48-1992 (Permanence of Paper)

Cover photo of Borden Flats "Lighthome," Fall River, MA, by Kevin Ferias, www.bordenflats.com

Photo of Mary Sullivan, courtesy of Mary Sullivan

"I Want to Age Like Sea Glass," reprinted with permission by Bernadette Noll

This book is dedicated
to the men and women
who have devoted their lives
to working in the field of nursing.
They are truly the backbone
of the medical profession.

Contents

Acknowledgments

I wish to recognize the following hospitals for their exemplary nursing care, which I have witnessed personally:

Yale New Haven Hospital
Backus Hospital
Pequot Medical Center
St. Ann's Hospital

I am grateful to the following people for the various ways they have supported my emotional, physical, spiritual, and professional well-being:

Beth Campbell
Bridget Henry
Clementine Thomas
Davin Michael Stedman
Debbie Chasen
Derrick Williams
Don Smead
Doug Knowlton
Glenn Linder
Jodi Purdy
Joe Agnello
Judy Bouley, CSA
Lisa Iannone Miller
Mike Panus
Naomi La Salsera Judia
Neil Hoss, DMD
Nicole Cassarino-Conlon
Northwell Health Nurse Choir
Ryan Kristafer

Sally Nasatka
Savinia Neal
Tina Maria Kiniry
Zandi Mbele

I am deeply grateful to the following writers, celebrities, and leaders, whose quotes have inspired inner strength in me:

A.A. Milne
Albert Camus
Albert Schweitzer
Alexander Graham Bell
Alfa
Amanda Gorman
Andy Rooney
Anuj Setia
Arlin Sailesh Kapadia
Aryn Kyle
Barack Obama
Becca Anderson
Bernadette Noll
Bob Marley
Brandon Hatmaker
Brené Brown
Bronwyn Lea
Buddha
Carl Sagan
Dan Rather
Danielle Steel
David Ault
David Sarnoff
David Soul
Davin Michael Stedman
Deb Johnson
Debasish Mridha, M.D.
Denis Waitley
Dr. Daniel Milstein
Dr. Miguel Cardona
Dr. Seuss
Dr. Wayne W. Dyer
Edith Wharton
Germany Kent
Isaac Newton
Iyanla Vanzant
Jay Shetty
Joel Osteen
John C. Maxwell
John Muir
Jonathan Lockwood Huie
Joseph Joubert
Judy Collins
Juri Love
Kahlil Gibran
Katrina Mayer
Kristen Butler

Kurt Vonnegut
Laila Gifty Akita
Linjl Yixuan
Lisa Fantino
Marcus Terentius Varro
Mark Twain
Matshona T. Dhilwayo
Max Ehrmann
Maya Angelou
Mehmet Murat ildan
Melody Beattie
Michael Moore
Michelle Obama
Muhammad Ali
Nelson Rockefeller
Nipsey Hussle
Oprah Winfrey
Orebela Gbenga
Paolo Coelho
Queen Latifah
Rachel Marie Martin
Ralph Waldo Emerson
Ram Charan
Roald Dahl
Robert Louis Stevenson
Roger Lee
Roxana Jones
Roy Goodman
Roy T. Bennett
Rumi
RVM
S. Anja
S. R. Abbasi
Sandy Coleman
Sarah Dessen
Shruti Gaja
Socrates
Soren Kierkegaard
Steven Fields
Sugar Ray Leonard
The Mindset Journey
Thomas Jefferson
Thomas S. Monson
Tim McGraw
Tom Hanks
Topher Pike
Vince Lombardi
Werner Erhard
William James
Yoko Ono
Zhuangzi
Ziad Abdelnour
Zig Ziglar

Foreword

A Nurse's Story

Mary Sullivan, MSN, RNC-MNN

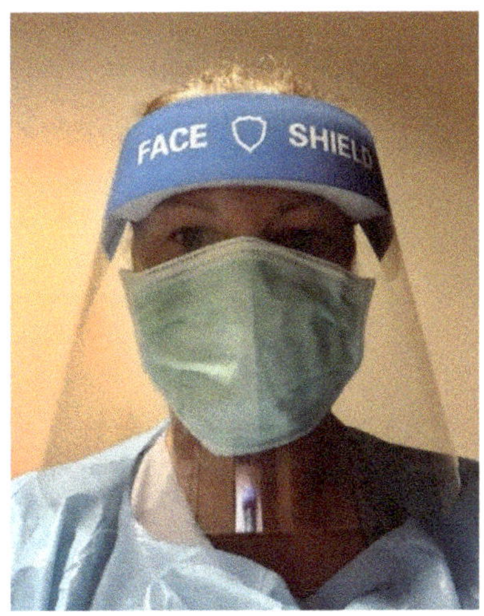

This beautifully written book, *Finding Peace by the Sea*, is a true gift of light to humanity, especially for people like me, who continue to be faced with the unthinkable during this ongoing pandemic. I have found renewed personal strength in reading it. It has shed a guiding light on my path in these difficult times. I have embraced many of Harry's principles for living your best life, namely, keeping a strong work ethic, maintaining an attitude of gratitude and humility, having the courage to step out of my comfort zone, and staying focused on my purpose of serving others.

As the mother of nine children, a registered nurse, nurse educator and mental health nurse practitioner student, I am grateful to God for the serenity I am able to access each time I visit the seaside. The peace I find by the sea has played a vital role in my journey of self-love and healing at times when I was feeling most overwhelmed. For me, the seaside is a potent remedy to the stress and chaos of everyday life. Harry Thomas shares this powerful coping strategy in his book, along with his own twelve personal principles for living his best life. Harry's book offers hope and guidance to those who are overwhelmed and have lost their direction due to unforeseen life events.

On January 24, 2019, Martin Joseph Sullivan, the father of my nine children suffered a fatal heart attack. The shock and devastation were immeasurable because he was 57 years old and perceived to be in decent health. The ocean remained my escape—it's where I go to find refuge and to de-stress. I took many beach walks and prayed for strength to help my children get through this tragic event. I prayed that I would have the courage to stand in front of my nursing students and deliver effective lectures on pharmacology, which included teaching about medications given to prevent heart disease and heart attacks. My Maternal Newborn lectures were triggering as I spoke about new life coming into the world since Marty and I shared that experience nine times.

Just after the one-year anniversary of Marty's death, I was back at the hospital working my second job. I was a bedside nurse while still teaching full-time at the college, and the Covid-19 pandemic was raging. This was a time of sheer uncertainty and more stress. In the Mother Infant Unit, where I worked every Friday and Saturday night, we had to separate newborns from the Covid-positive mothers as soon as they were born. The nurses took turns caring for either the mother or the baby while wearing personal protective equipment (PPE) for 12+ hours. After stressful hospital shifts, I would again go to the ocean to find peace and strength.

I don't share my story for sympathy because I understand that everyone has their own story of pain and suffering. My hope is that when you are faced with the unthinkable, you will find an outlet to help you cope. To all my fellow healthcare workers around the world, always stay mindful of your mental health and take the time to decompress. It is imperative!

I find Harry Thomas' creativity with the way he pairs beautiful photographs and meaningful quotes to be a gem that has both inspired and given me renewed hope.

Mary Sullivan, MSN, RNC-MNN

Introduction

As I watch the sun set each night over the ocean, I truly marvel at the majesty of God's creation. We have been graced with the beauty of the local coastline. As a photographer, I have sought to capture the space where Heaven and Earth intersect. Landscape is a universal expression of beauty, from the soothing blues of the water to the fiery color of the sunset. I have found inspiration and renewal waiting for me, down by the sea. Peace awaits me down by the sea. Almost magically, I find a sense of calm when I am near the ocean. I routinely escape the stress of daily life by heading to the shoreline. There's a sense of deep renewal down by the sea that I have not found anywhere else.

The sea is always there waiting for me, like a best friend who always has time for me. The sea gives me comfort, inspiration and unconditional support. I always feel better when I breathe the soothing ocean air. Down by the sea, I lose myself and let go of the worries of the day. The movement of the water invites me to breathe, relax and decompress. The gentle lull of the waves become a shadow of my own breathing, guiding me into a new sense of calm. My tension melts away. Troubles diminish in this powerful ritual that grounds me. All is well when I am down by the sea.

As I hold my camera steady on the landscape, all is well with my soul. Sensations of perpetual movement, sound and scent surrounds me. I have arrived at my happy place. I realize how deeply I am loved, and that the universe is, in fact, conspiring in my favor. The beauty of the landscape is captured and preserved by my lens for all to enjoy. I capture, for you and me, an image now locked in time.

I am drawn to the sea because, like many of you, my soul yearns to feel free from the burdens of the day. I desire inner peace in a world that often feels chaotic. I crave the ability to breathe freely, for that is true freedom. I seek a sense of inner peace. I think we all do, and yet it eludes so many of us.

Motivational quotes have been my anchor. For several years, I have embraced a daily ritual of selecting an inspirational quote and pairing it with my one of my seaside photographs to motivate me throughout the day. These combinations have given me direction and could perhaps do the same for you. My quote selections focus around twelve principles I have identified for living my best life. My twelve principles have kept me grounded and focused in recent years. I illustrate them through select quotes paired with my photos. I started finding inspiration in quotes at an early age under the teaching style of my mother in raising her children.

I want all of you to have access to the sense of personal empowerment and encouragement I have found through my photo and quote combinations. Peace, comfort, hope and guidance are universally needed now, in a world so challenged with economic strife, racial tension and moral erosion. We are in a society that craves stress relief but is so lacking in healthy coping skills. The universal need for stress relief inspired me to use my background as a mental health professional and educator to write my first book,

Peace by the Sea: Inspiring Images and Quotes to Light Your Way.

I was compelled to write another book upon hearing from readers that *Peace by the Sea* has been bringing comfort and peace to people suffering from anxiety, stress, grief, trauma, relationship issues, and economic insecurity. As a mental health professional, I recognize the need for peace in the world and humbly offer my own personal wisdom. My twelve principles for living my best life offer guidance for staying grounded and motivated.

In *Finding Peace by the Sea*, I bring the serenity of the New England seaside to you, paired with select quotes. I share my photo-quote combinations to uplift others. My intention is that you will be inspired and encouraged. I achieve a sense of inner peace by living by these twelve guiding principles:

- ❖ Peace is keeping a humble perspective by focusing on the bigger picture. It's not all about me.
- ❖ Peace is maintaining an attitude of gratitude and expressing appreciation to others where it is due.
- ❖ Peace is recognizing and embracing the strength and personal power that is within us.
- ❖ Peace is found through self-reflecting, which is the root to strong character.
- ❖ Peace is being courageous enough to step out of the comfort zone and seize the opportunities that life has to offer.

- ❖ Peace is finding direction and purpose and walking that path confidently.
- ❖ Peace is embracing my responsibilities with a strong work ethic.
- ❖ Peace is accepting the challenge of obstacles and creatively identifying strategies for overcoming them.
- ❖ Peace is trusting my intuition when making tough decisions, recognizing that the answer lies within me.
- ❖ Peace is nurturing positive social connections and letting go of toxic ones.
- ❖ Peace is opening your heart and being willing to be vulnerable and authentic.
- ❖ Peace is found by being one with nature. Peace is within reach down by the sea.

I am grateful to impart my humble wisdom to you. Perhaps one of my quote selections will become a mantra for your daily self-reflection and personal empowerment. As you look at these photographs and read these quotes, let yourself escape the troubles of the day. Imagine that you are there, in the scene of the photo. Inhale the peace that you need. Exhale the fear that stops you from living your best life. Inhale strength. Exhale the weight of all that burdens you. Let the peace of the sea replenish your soul. Be filled with gratitude for all that is good.

CHAPTER 1

Keeping a Humble Perspective

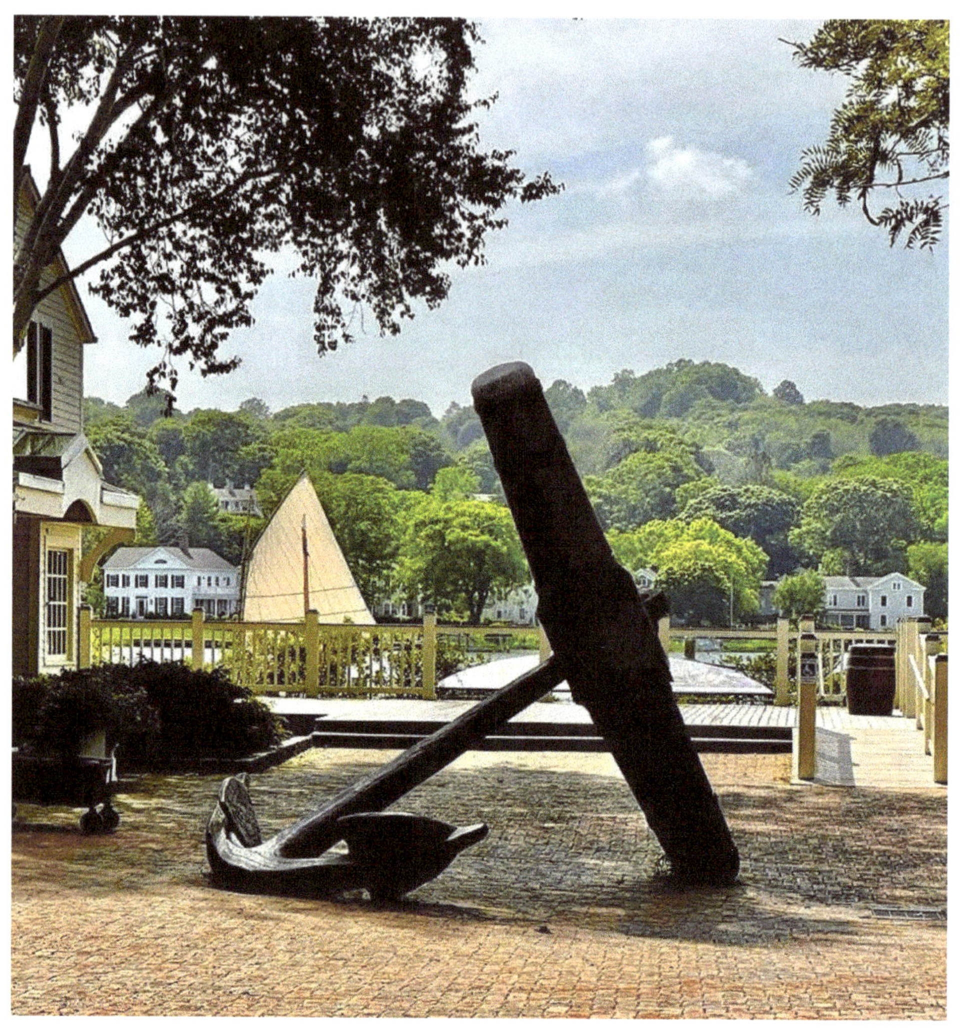

Faith gives us strength.
Grace gives us power.
Hope gives us anchor.

—Laila Gifty Akita

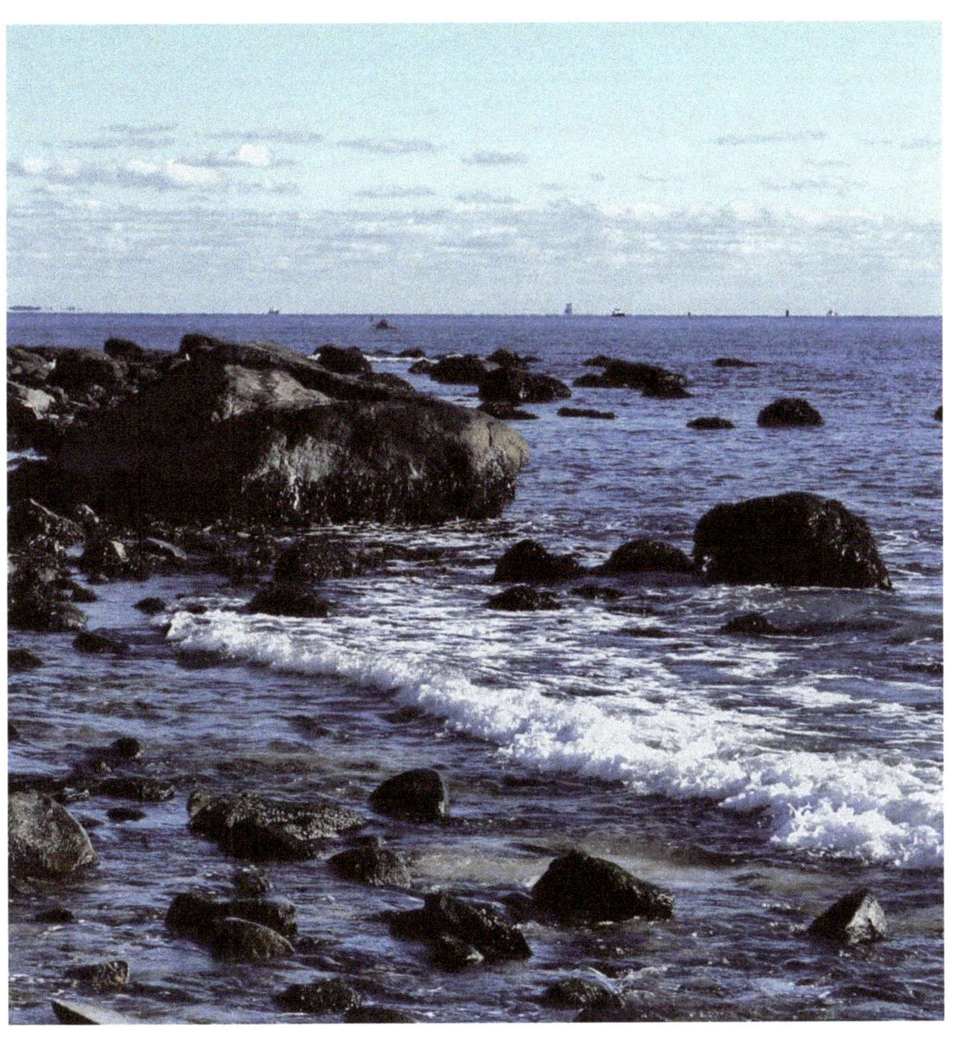

Remember there is no such thing
as a small act of kindness.
Every act creates a ripple with no logical end.

—Roald Dahl

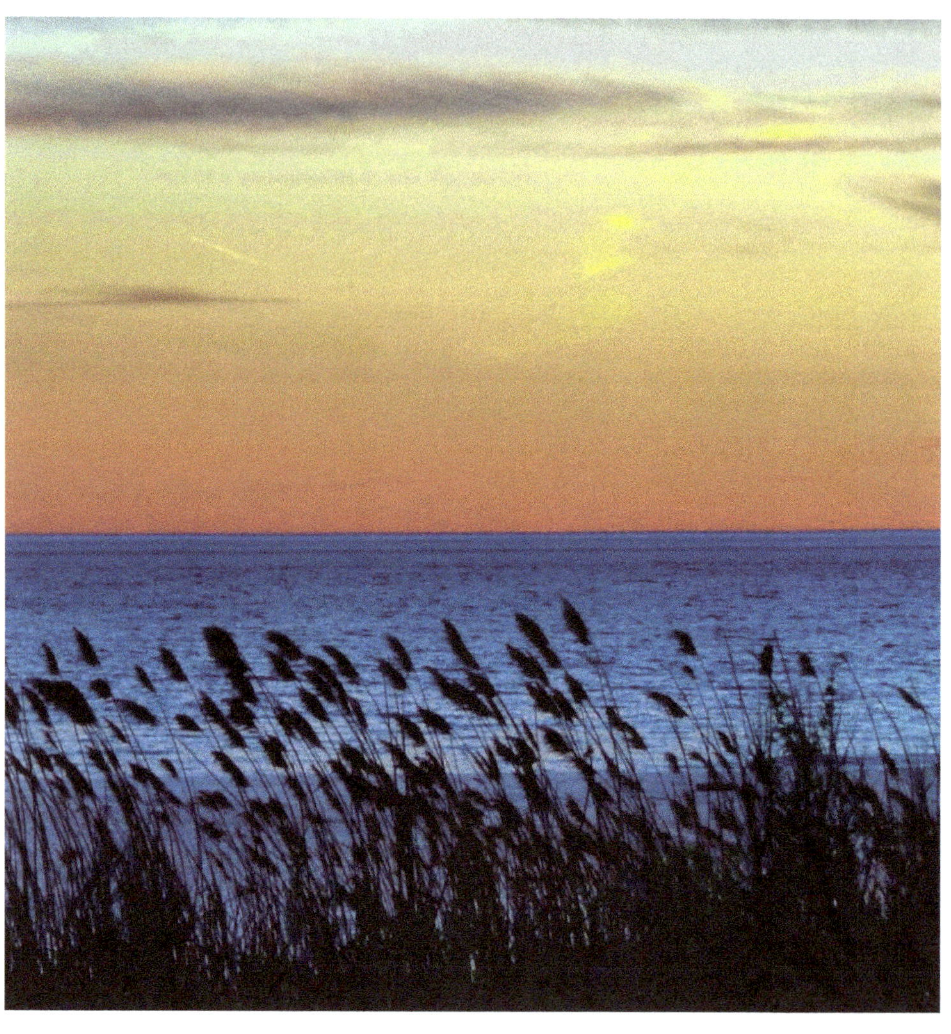

Never let success go to your head.
Never let failure get to your heart.

—Ziad Abdelnour

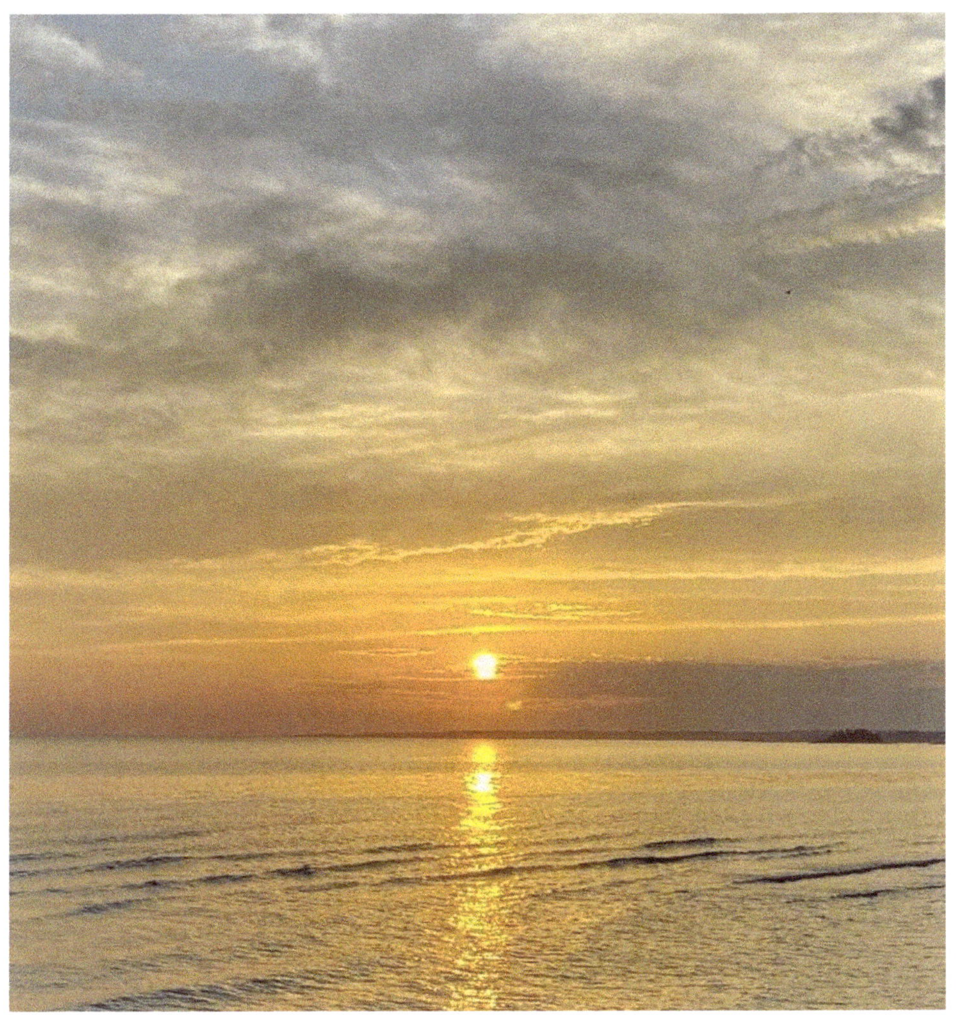

Enjoy the little things in life for one day you will look back and realize they were the big things.

—Kurt Vonnegut

Yesterday is history, tomorrow is a mystery,
but today is a gift.
That is why we call it The Present.

—A. A. Milne

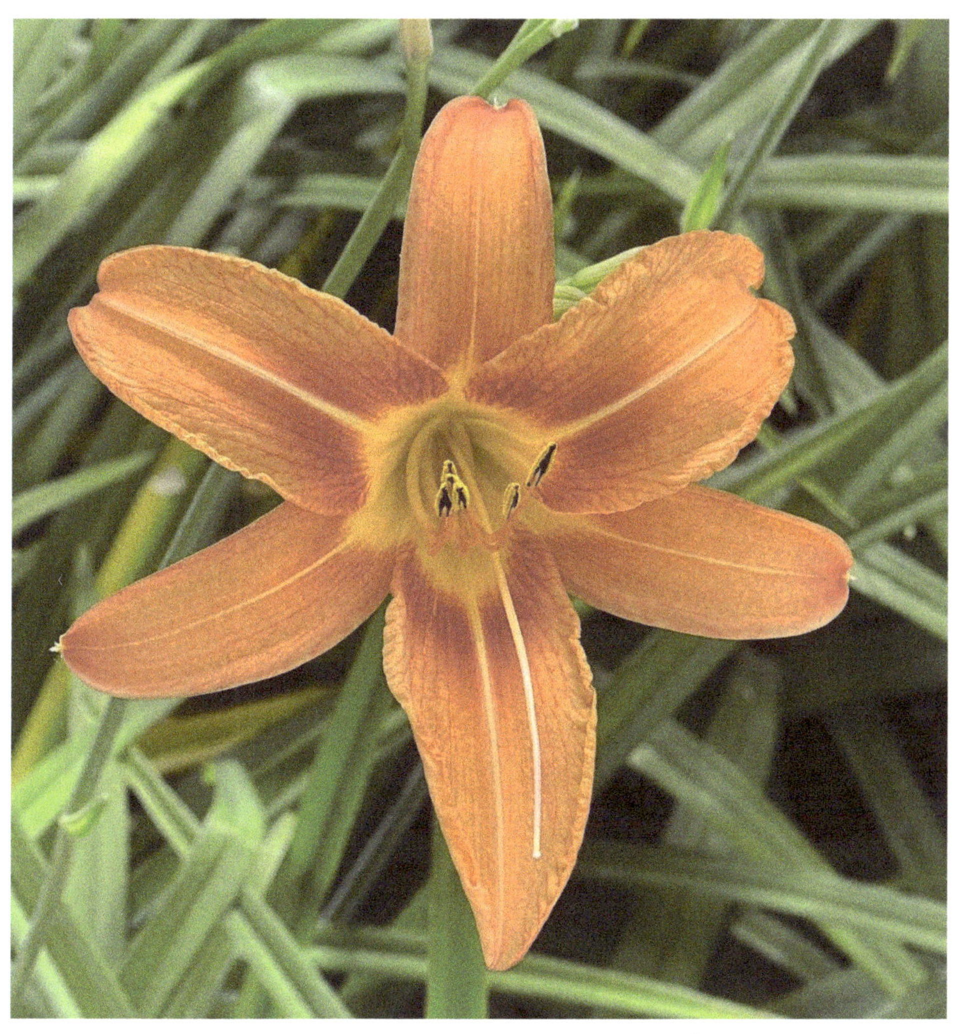

Politeness is the flower of humanity.

—Joseph Joubert

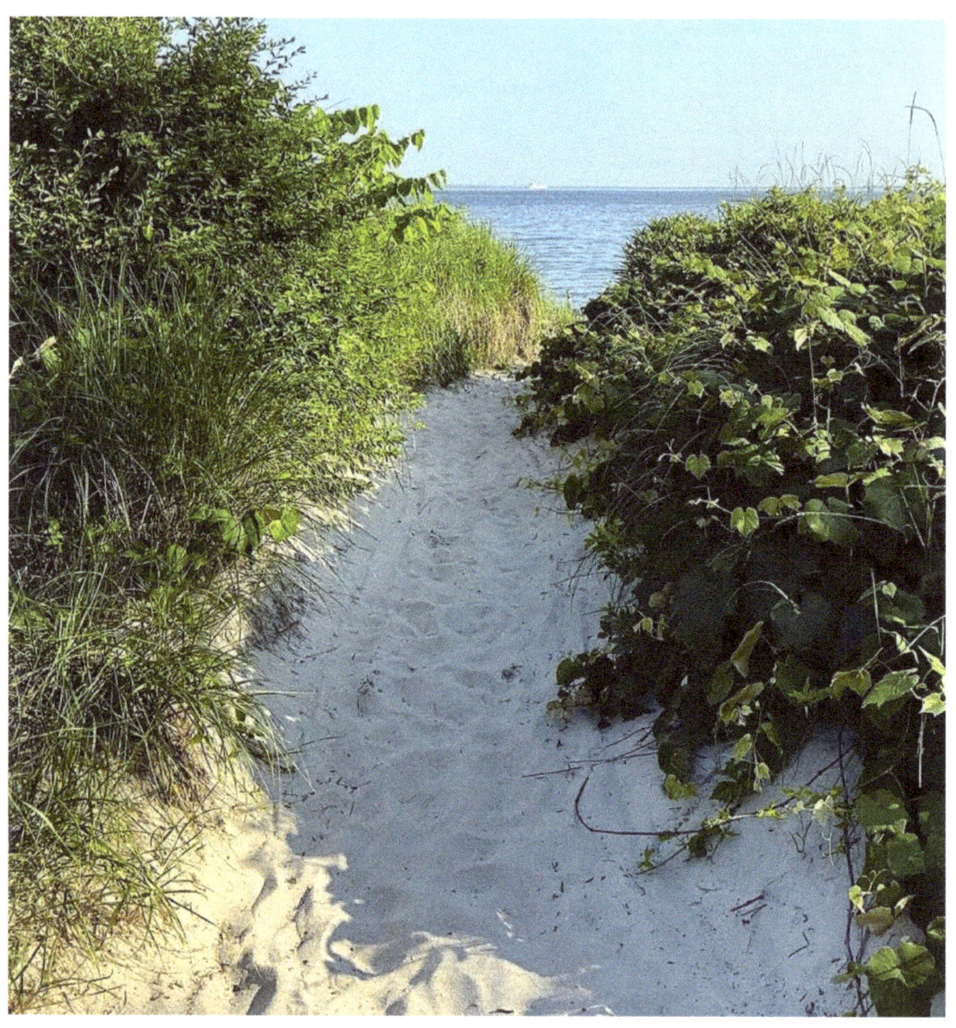

Travel the path of integrity without looking back,
for there is never a wrong time to do the right thing.

—Michael Moore

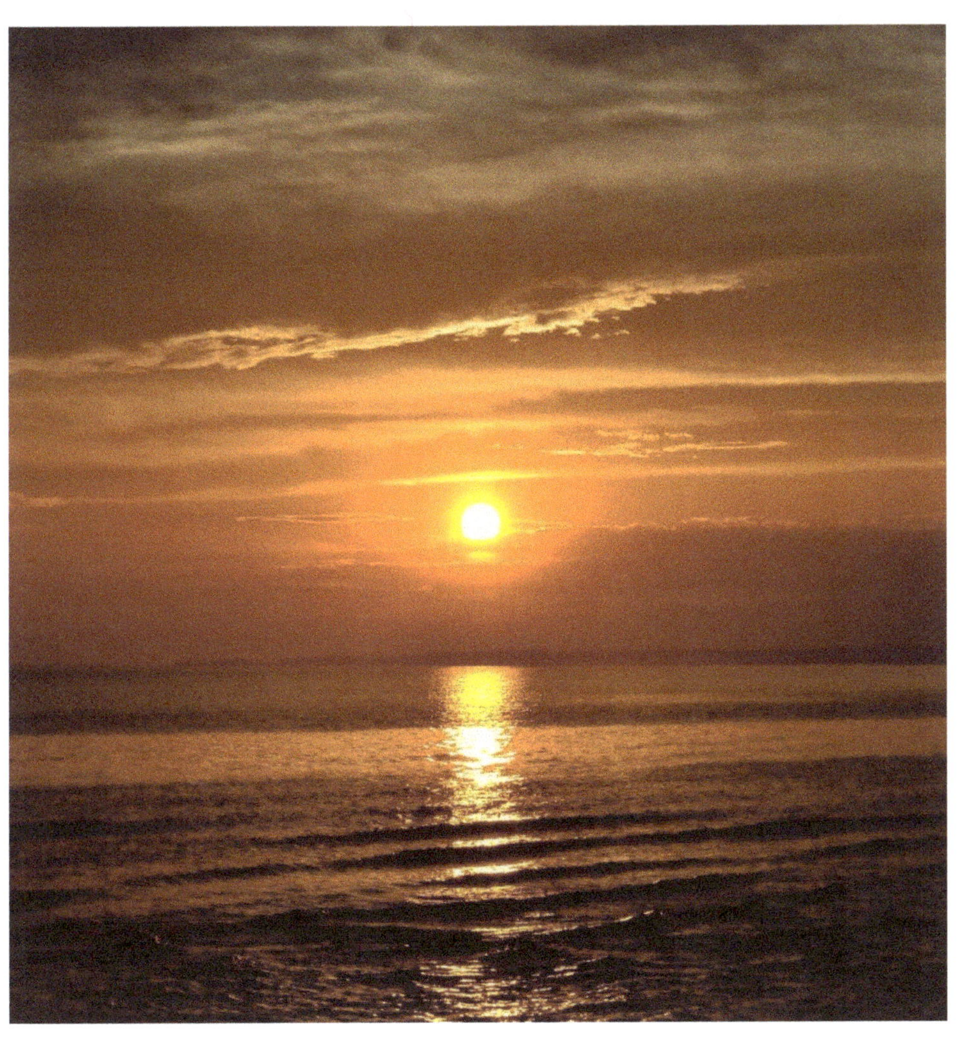

Don't wait for the perfect moment.
Take the moment and make it perfect!

—Aryn Kyle

CHAPTER 2

Being Grateful

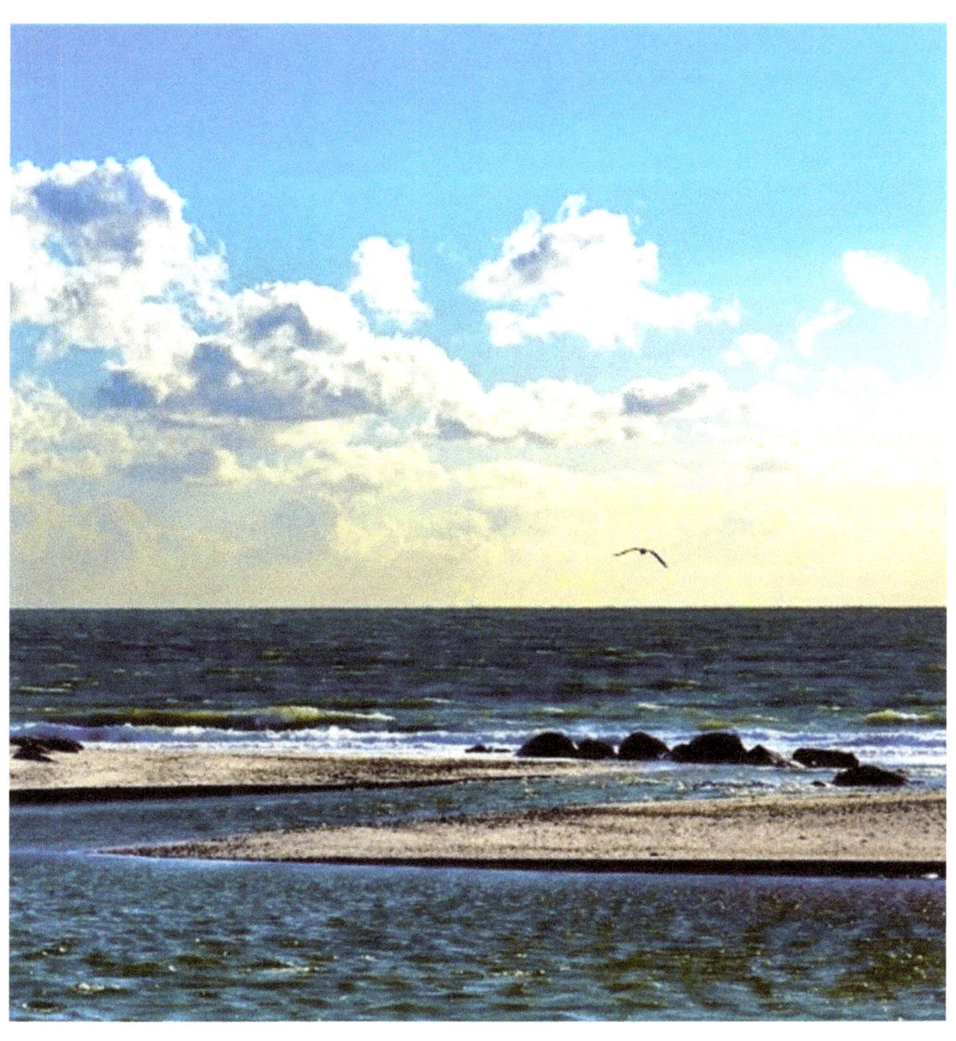

Happiness cannot be traveled to, owned, earned or consumed. Happiness is the spiritual experience of living every minute with love, grace, and gratitude.

—Denis Waitley

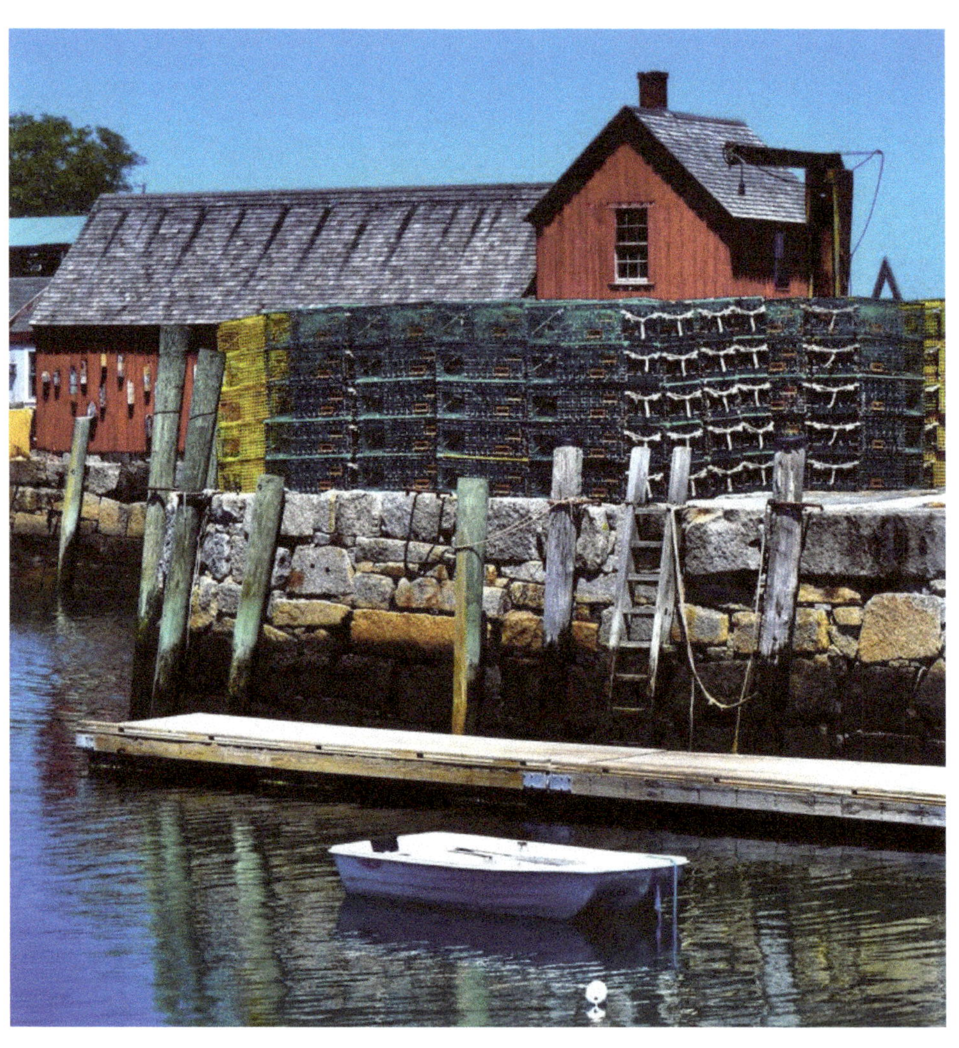

I've learned ....
That when you harbor bitterness,
happiness will dock elsewhere.

—Andy Rooney

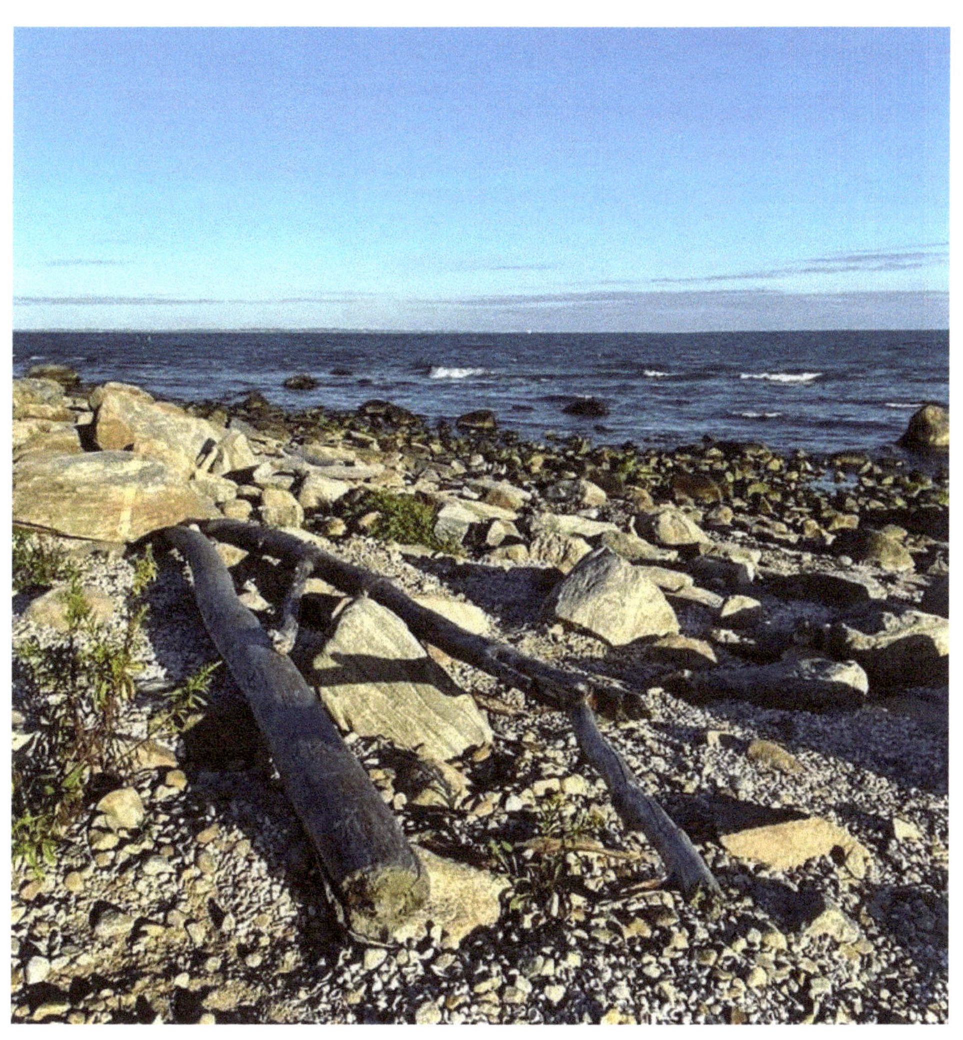

Love the life you live. Live the life you love.

—Bob Marley

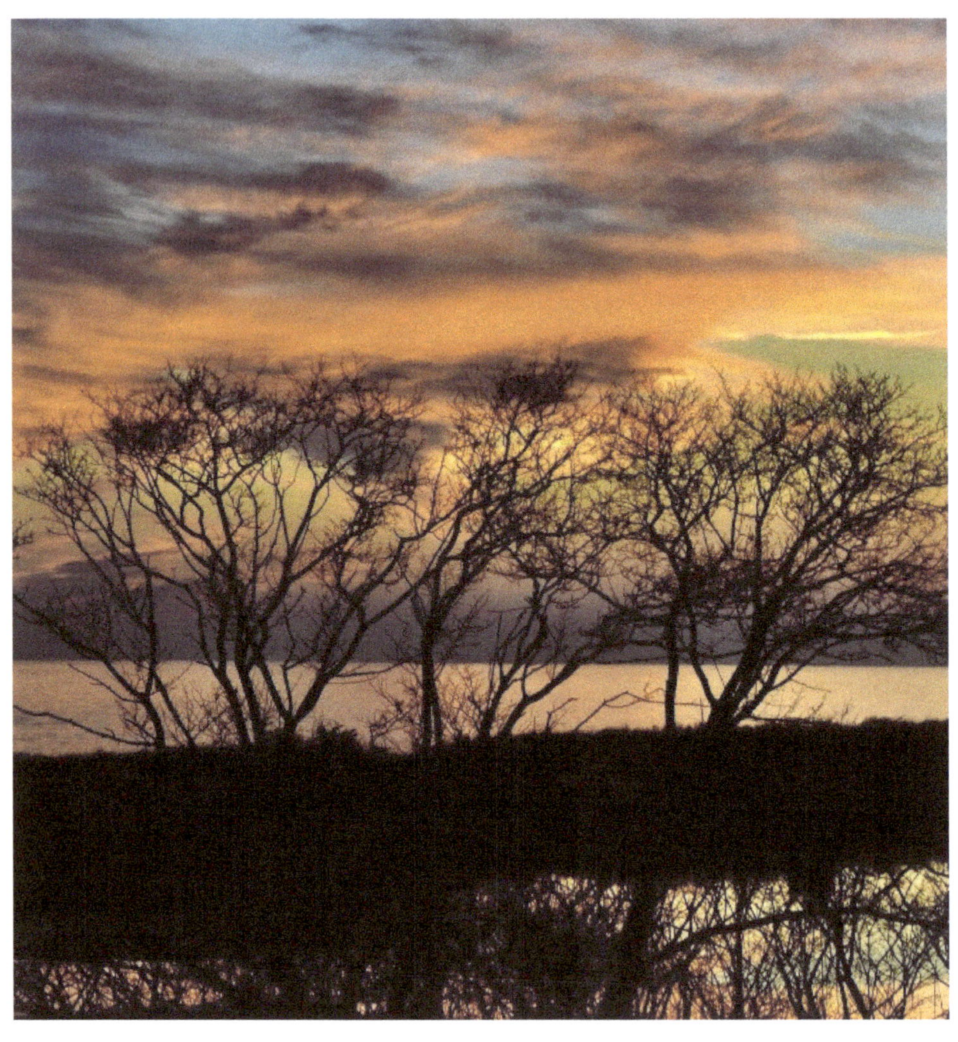

The sky speaks in a thousand colors.

—S. R. Abbasi

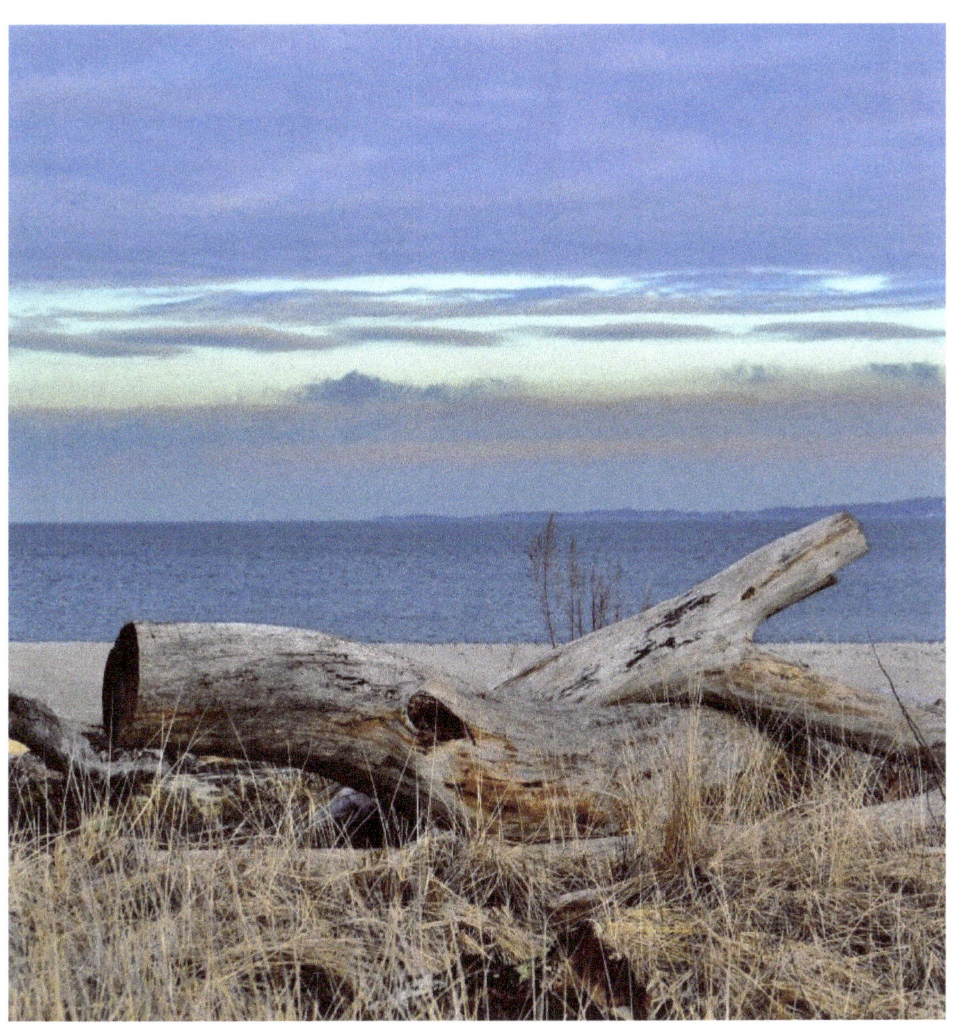

The happiest people don't have the best of everything. They make the best of everything!

—Unknown

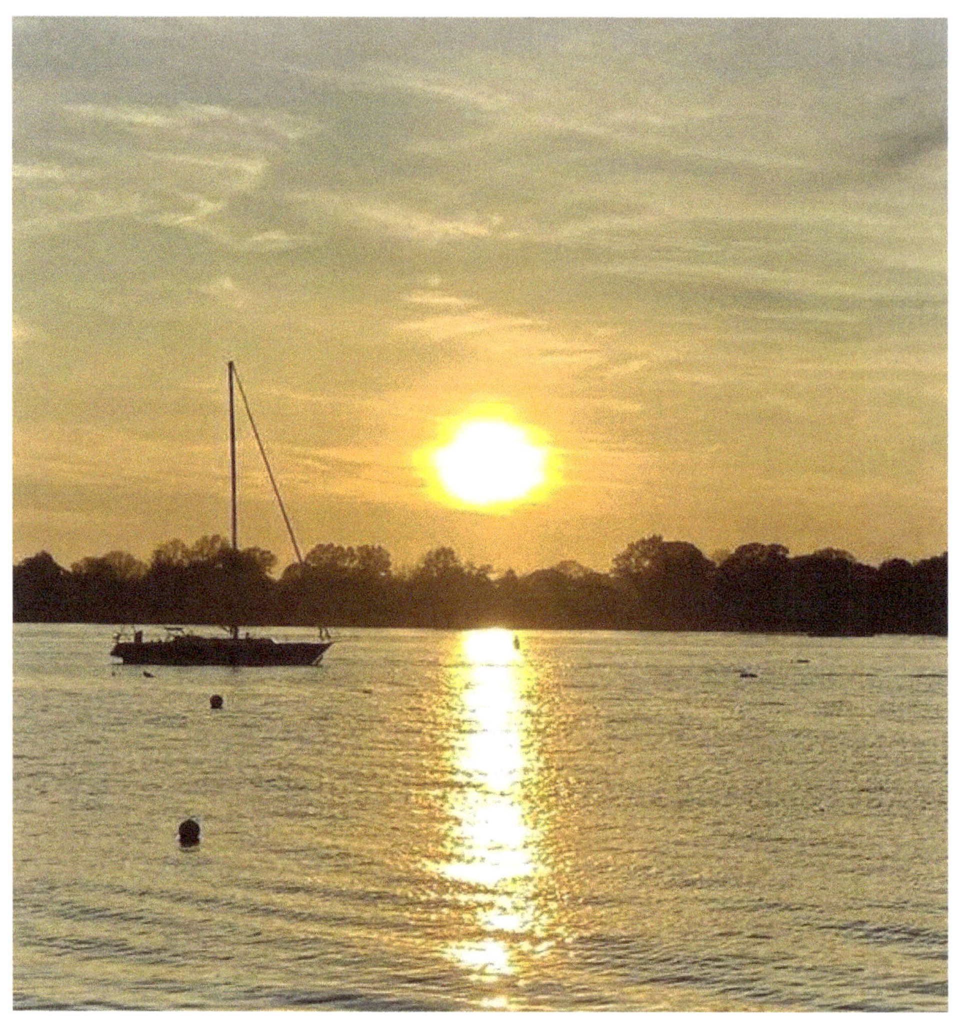

The main ingredients of happiness
are optimism and positivity.

—Juri Love

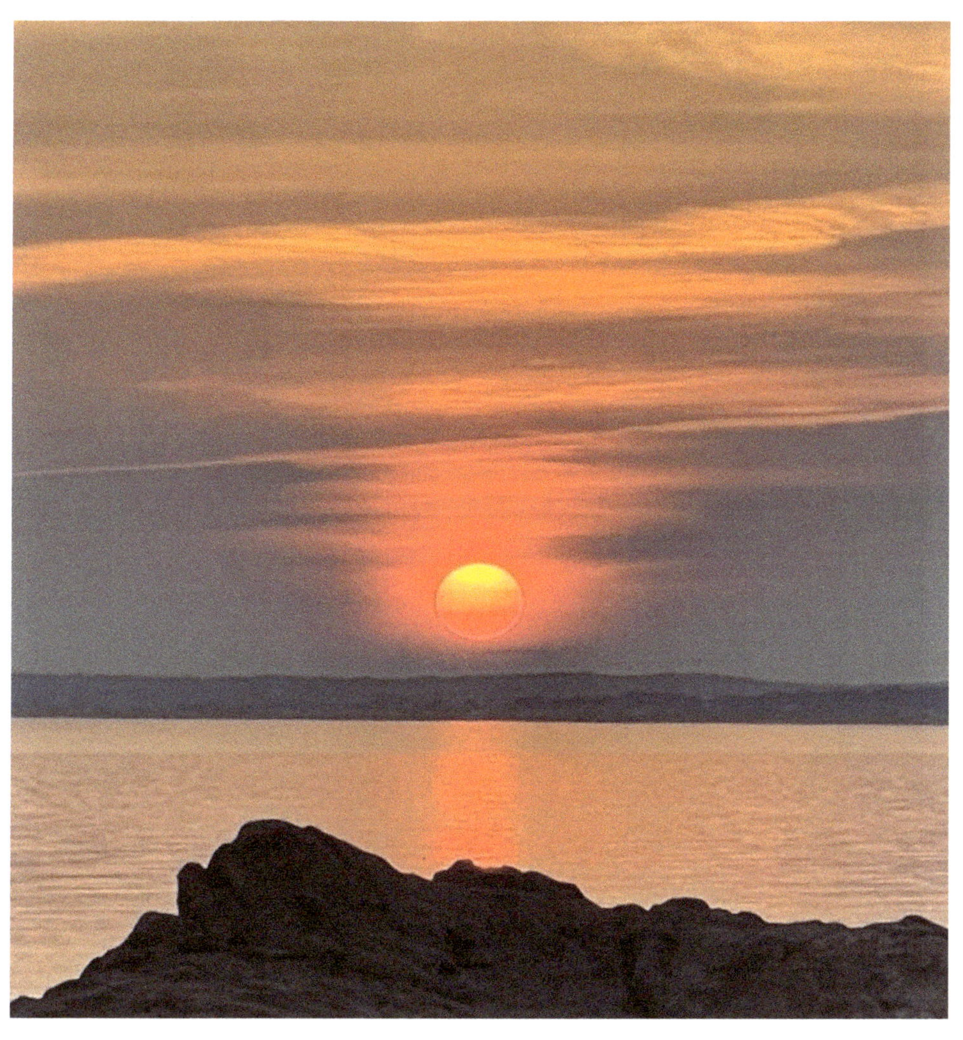

Let the fire in the sky light the fire in your soul.
Let the beauty all around you inspire you.

—Unknown

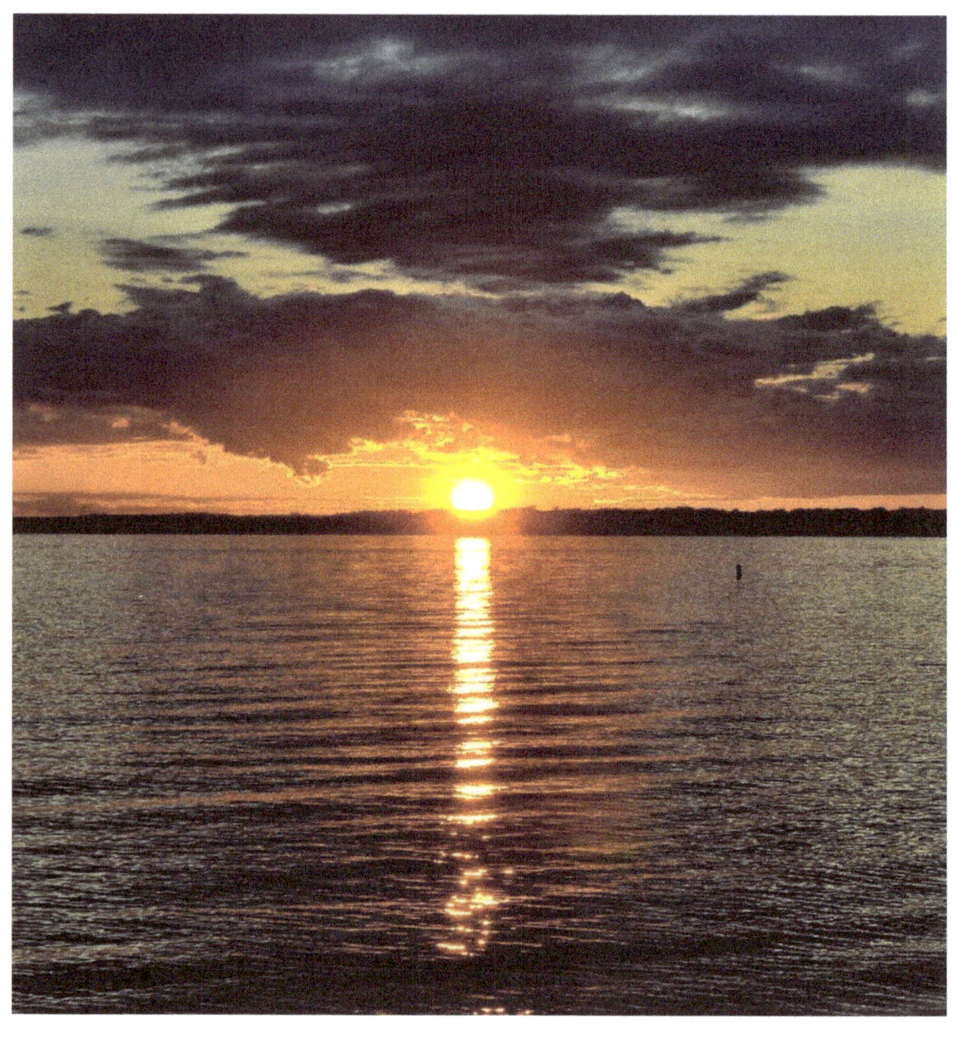

Sometimes you have to let go of the picture of
what you thought life would be like and learn
to find the joy in the story you are actually living.

—Rachel Marie Martin

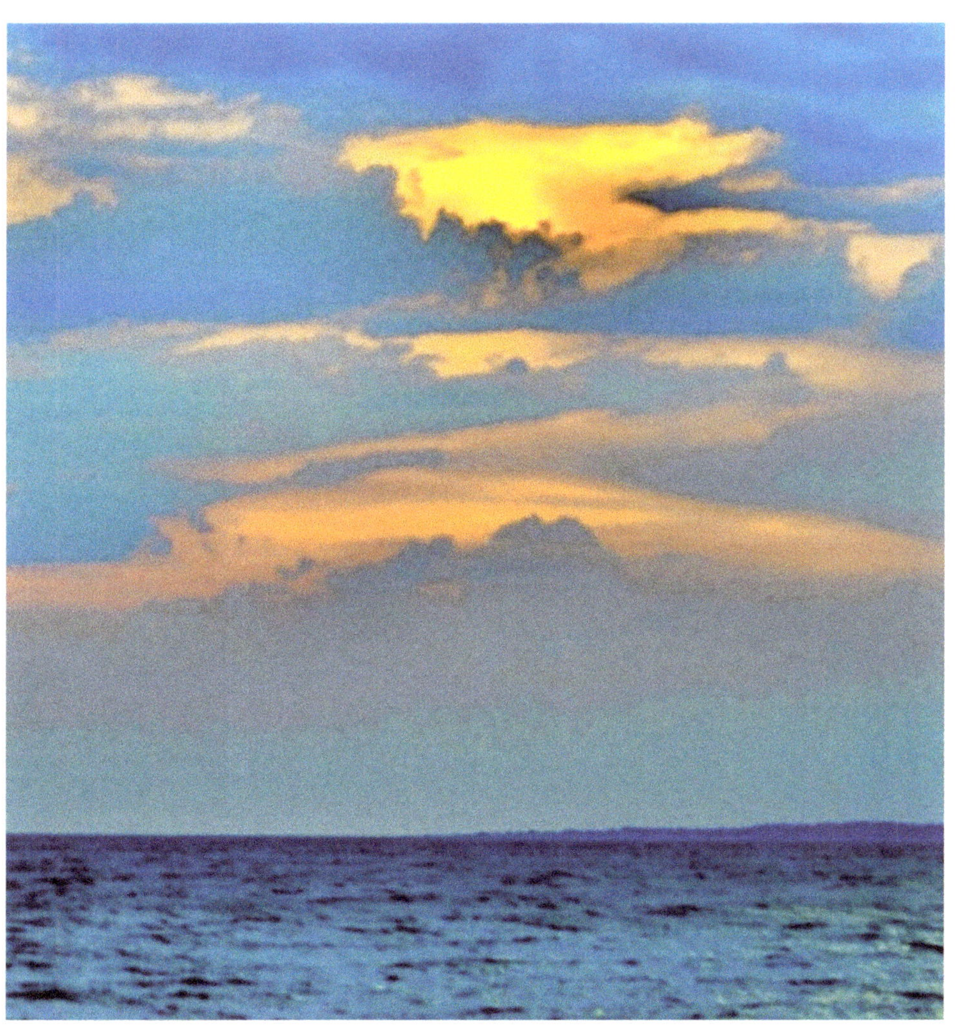

The truth about forever is
that it is happening right now.

—Sarah Dessen

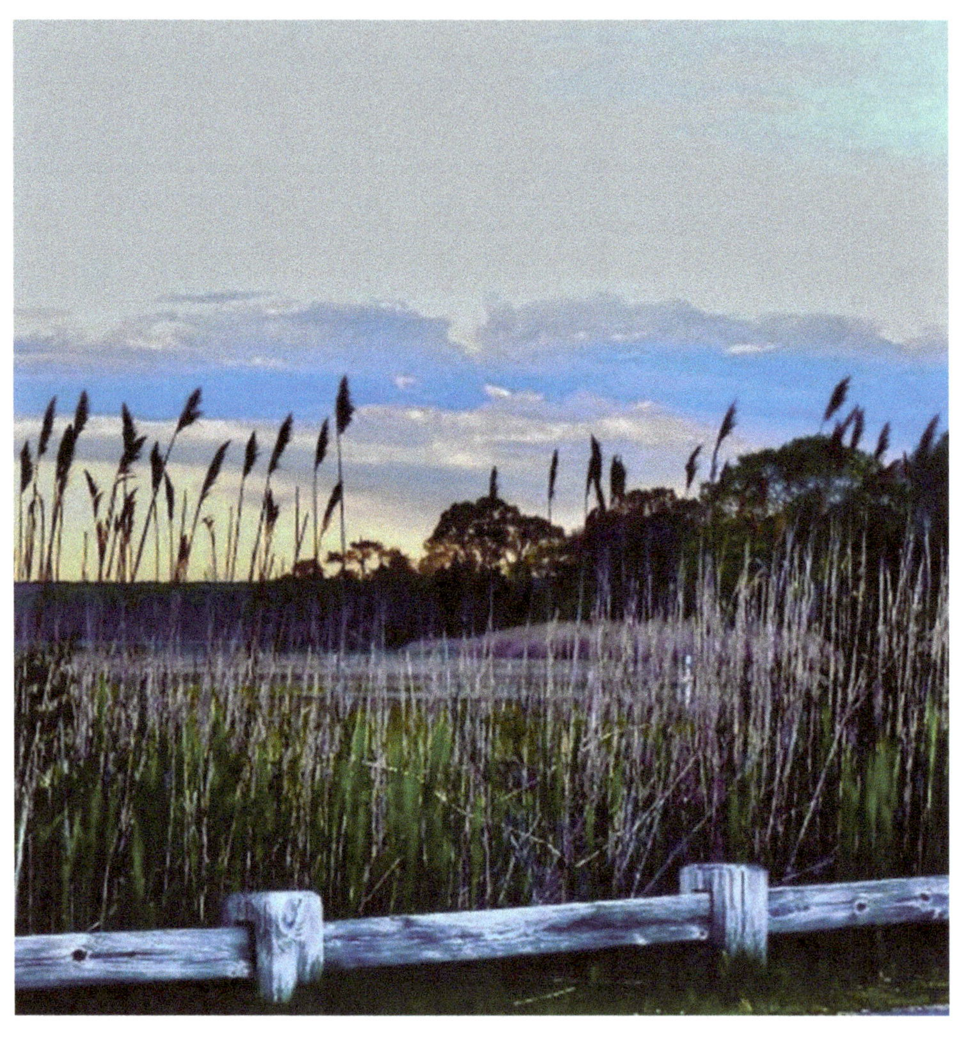

Gratitude makes sense of your past,
brings peace for today,
and creates a vision for tomorrow.

—Melody Beattie

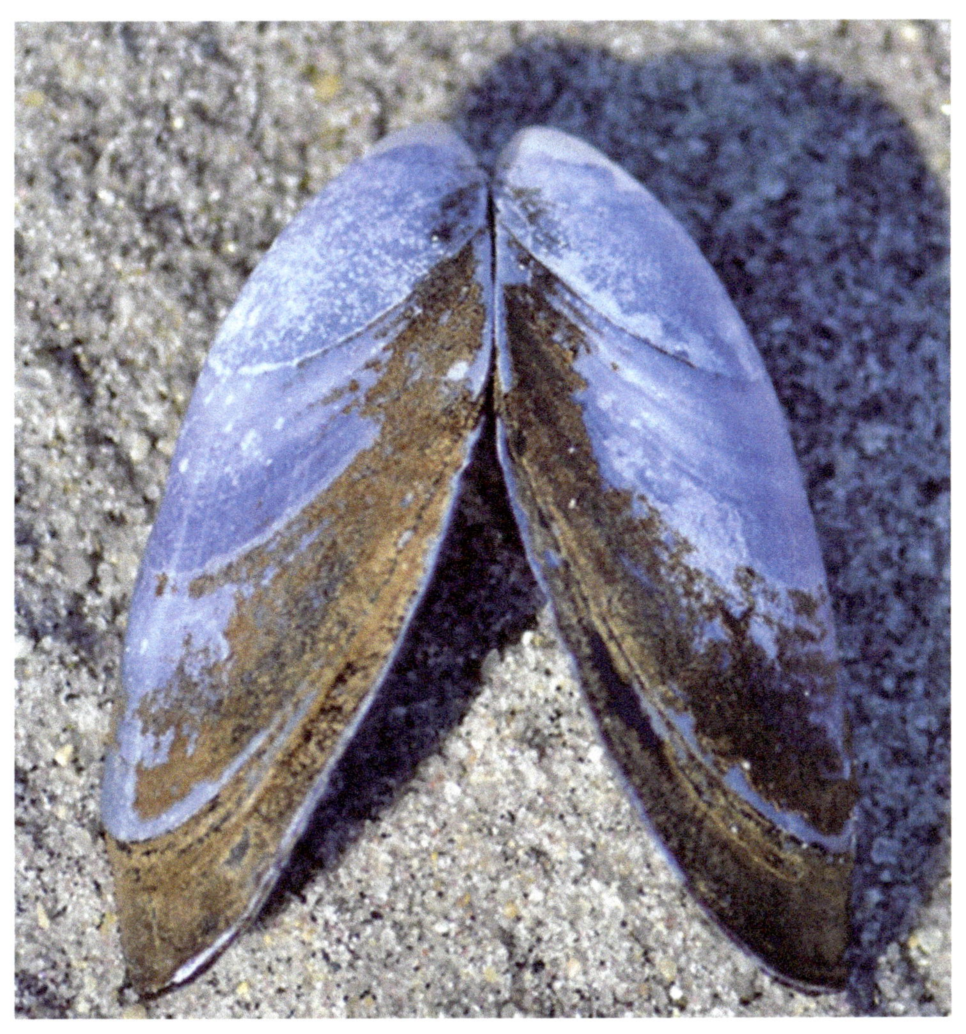

The measure of who we are is
what we do with what we have.

—Vince Lombardi

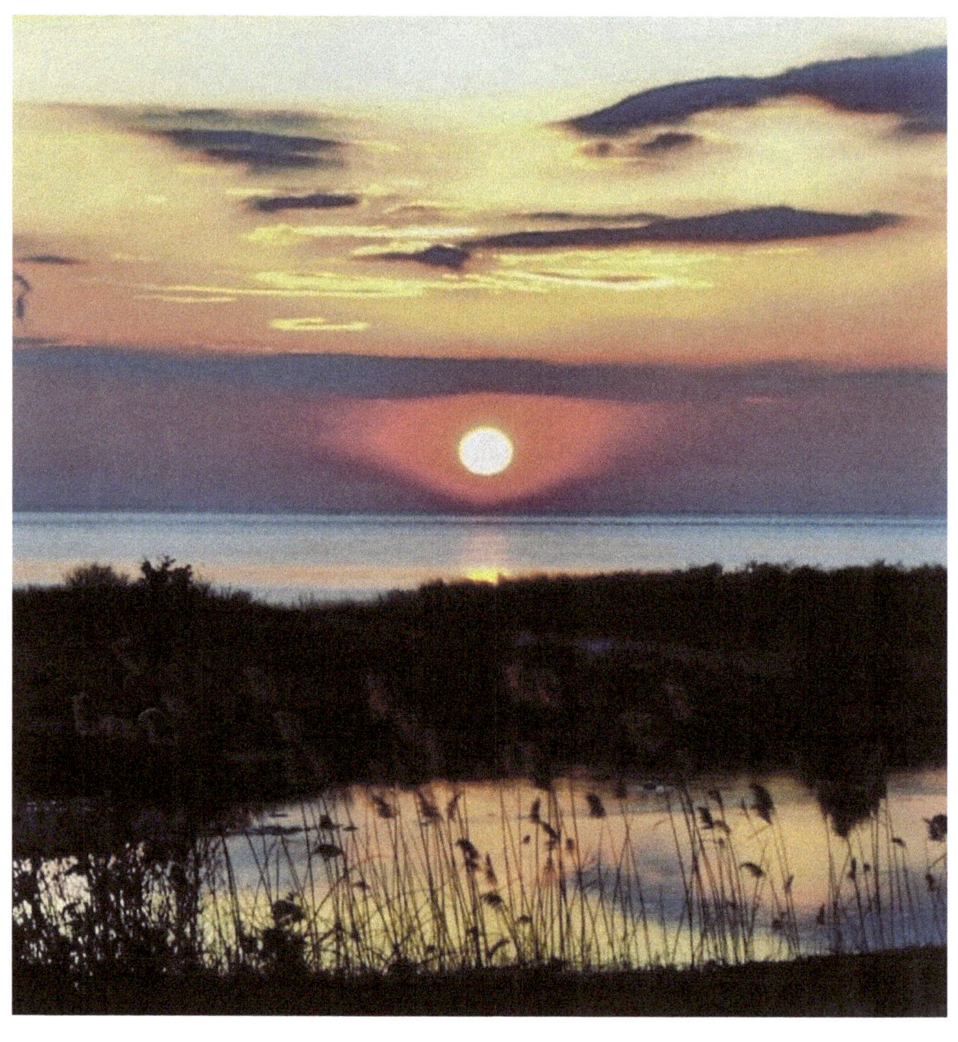

Sunsets are proof that no matter what happens,
everyday can end up beautifully.

—Kristen Butler

CHAPTER 3

Seizing Your Own Power

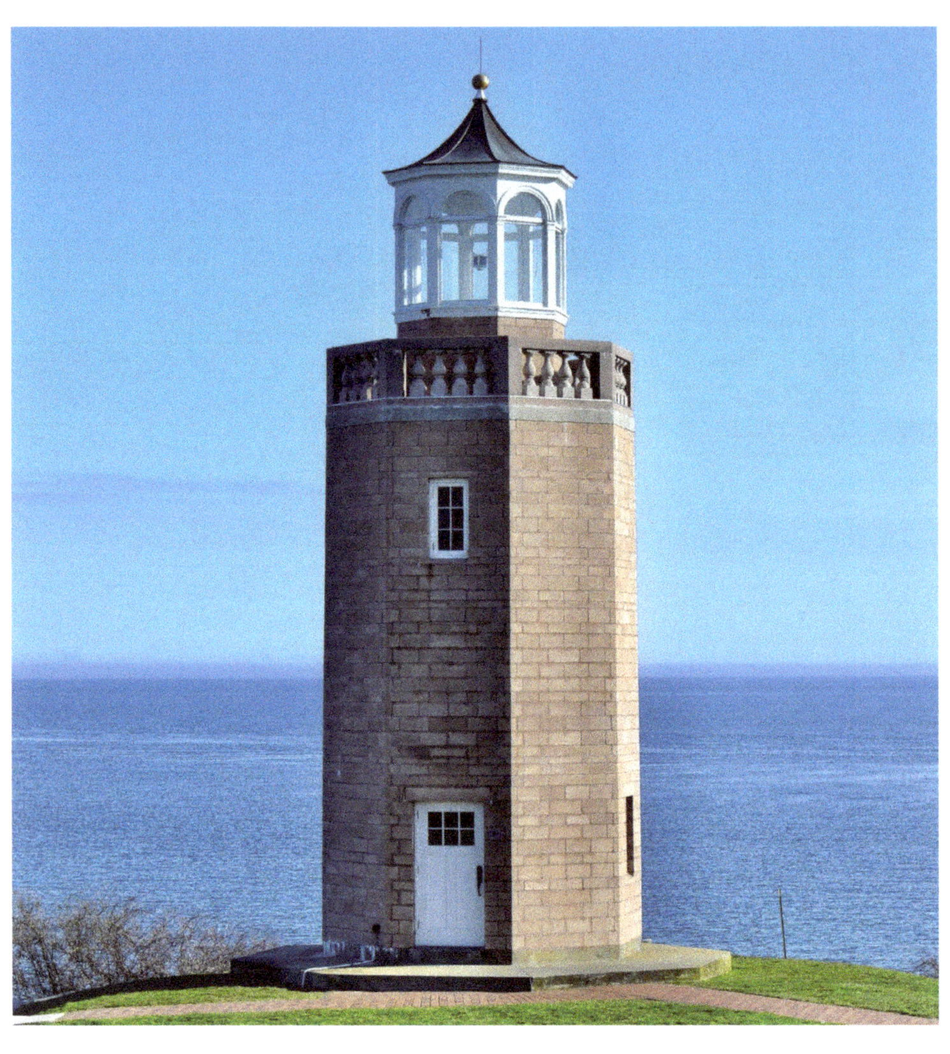

Be a lighthouse.
Shine for others whey they are in darkness.

—Unknown

If my mind can conceive it
and my heart can believe it,
I can achieve it.

—Muhammad Ali

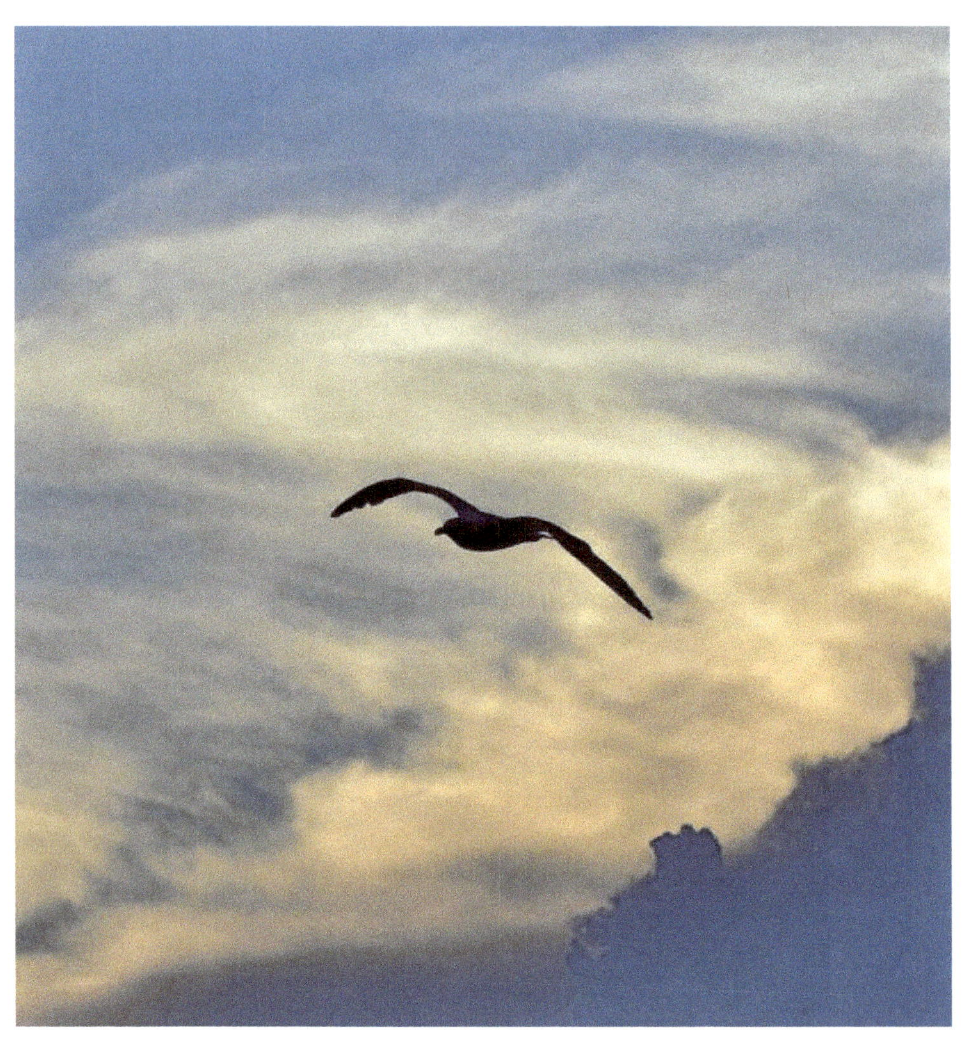

Become like a bird, expand your wings,
learn new things,
and fly as high as you can.

—Unknown

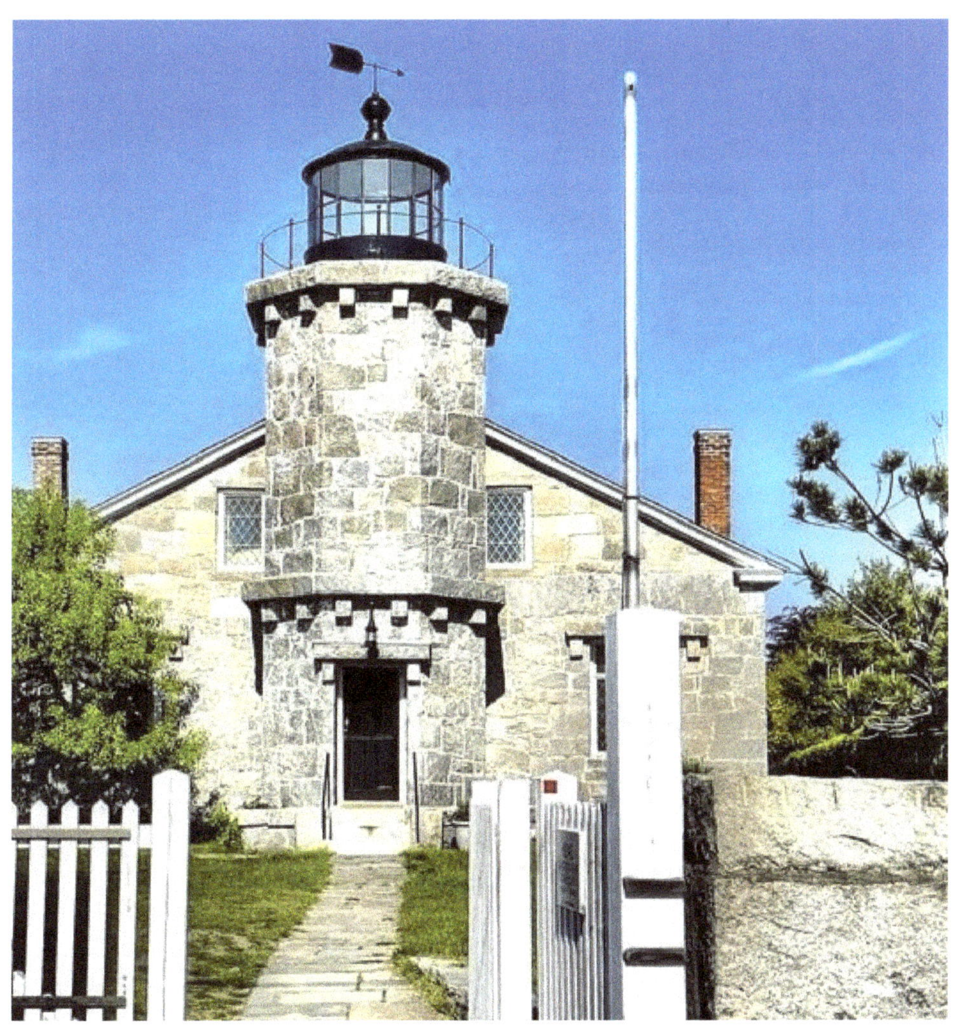

Nothing can dim the light that shines from within.

—Maya Angelou

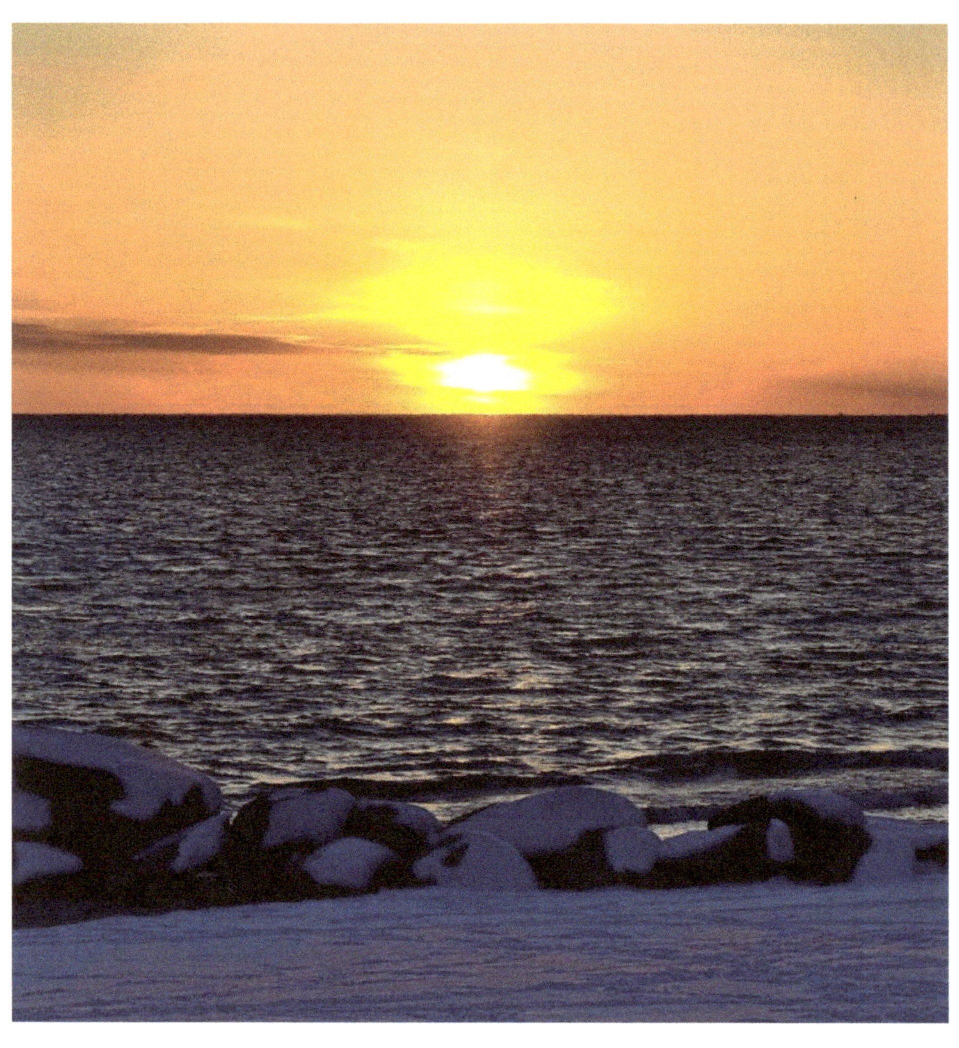

In the midst of winter,
I found there was, within me,
an invincible summer.

—Albert Camus

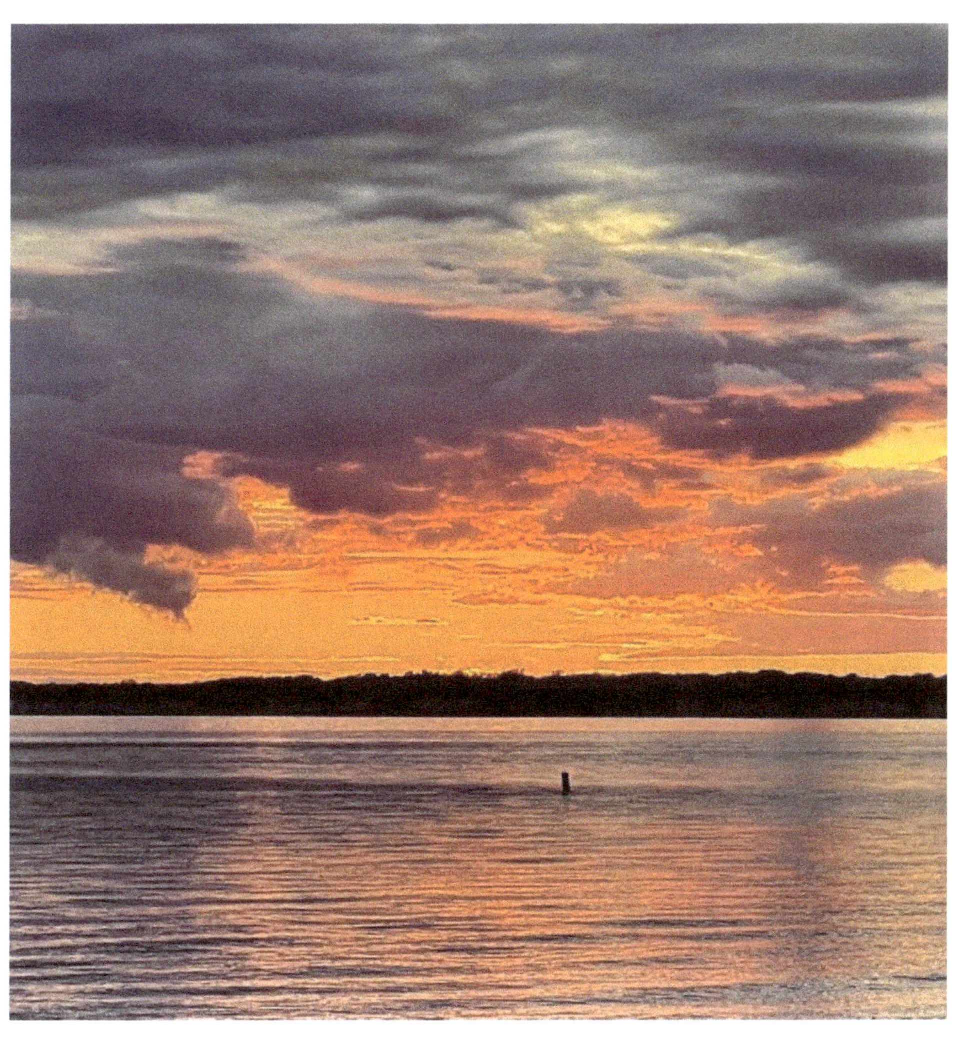

Don't wait for a storm to change your life;
create the storm that will change your life.

—Topher Pike

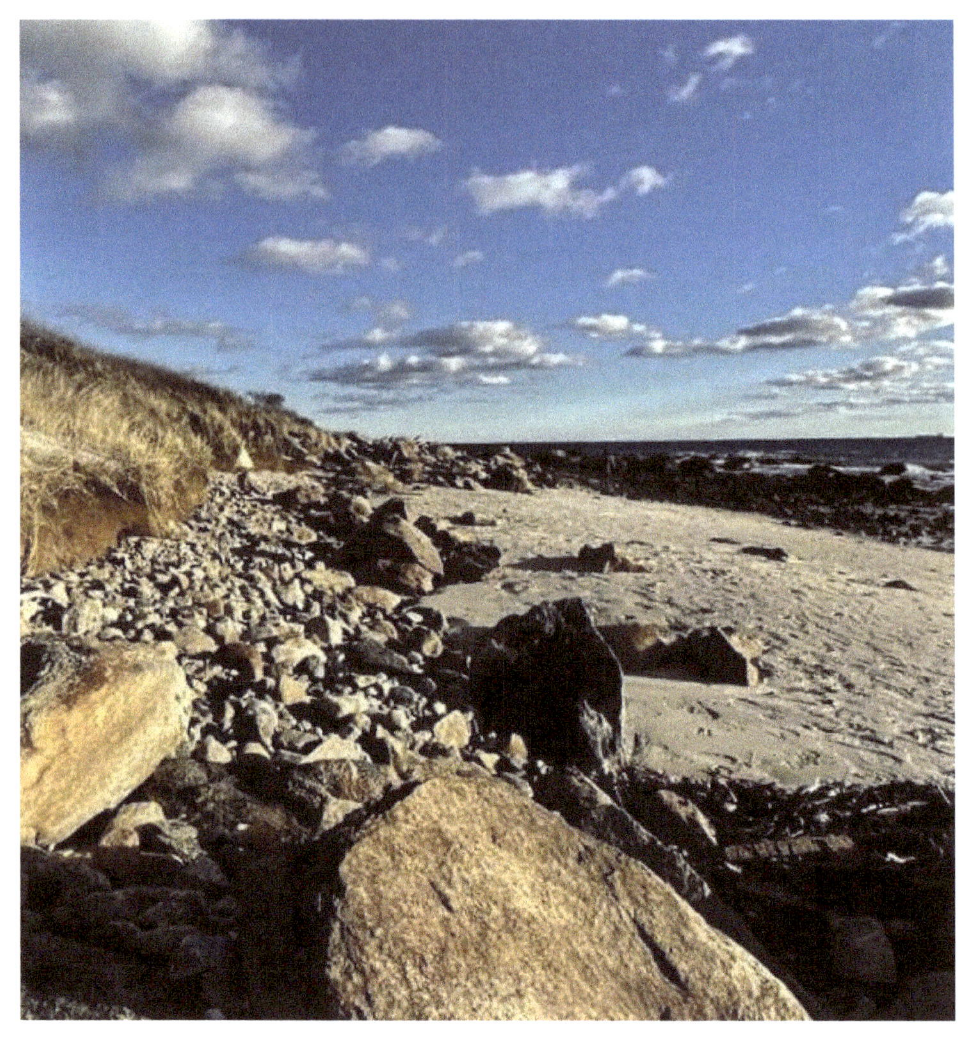

Act as if what you do makes a difference.
It does.

—William James

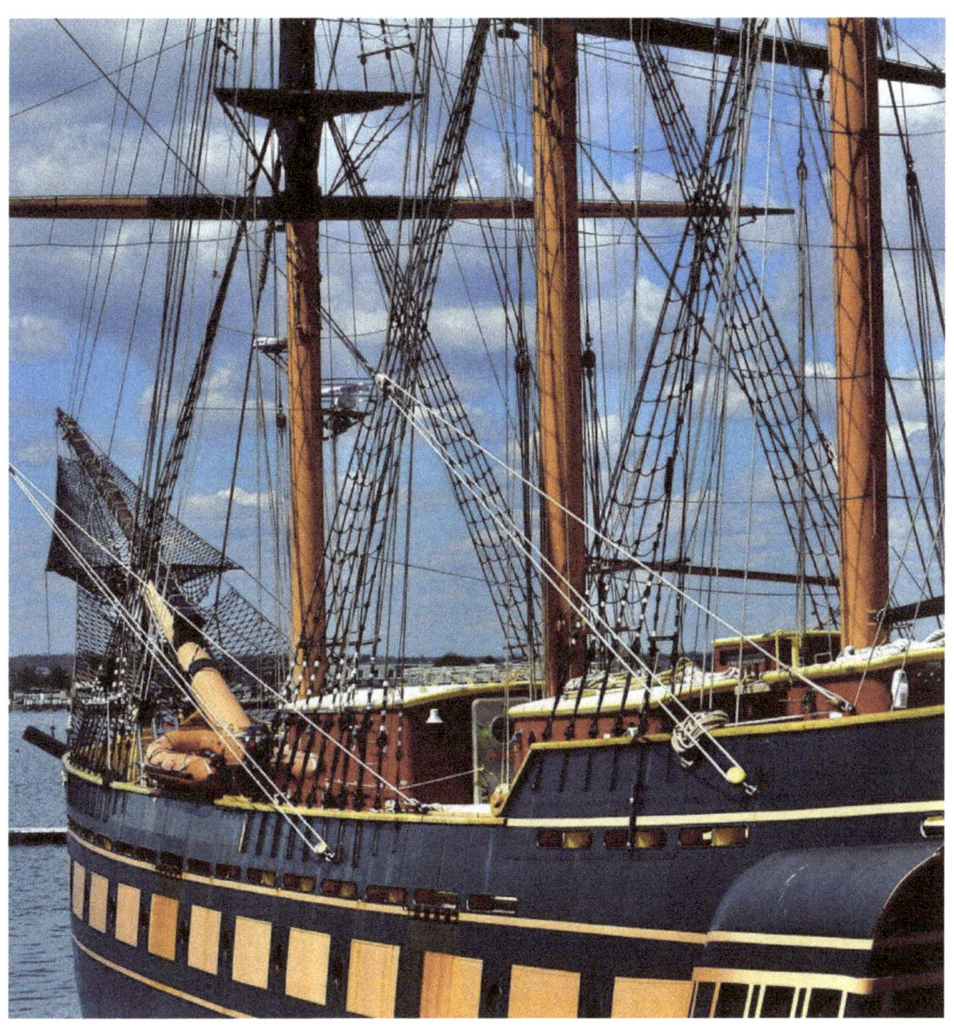

Twenty years from now, you will be more disappointed by the things you didn't do than those you did. So throw off the bowlines. Sail away from safe harbor. Catch the wind in your sails. Explore. Dream. Discover.

—Mark Twain

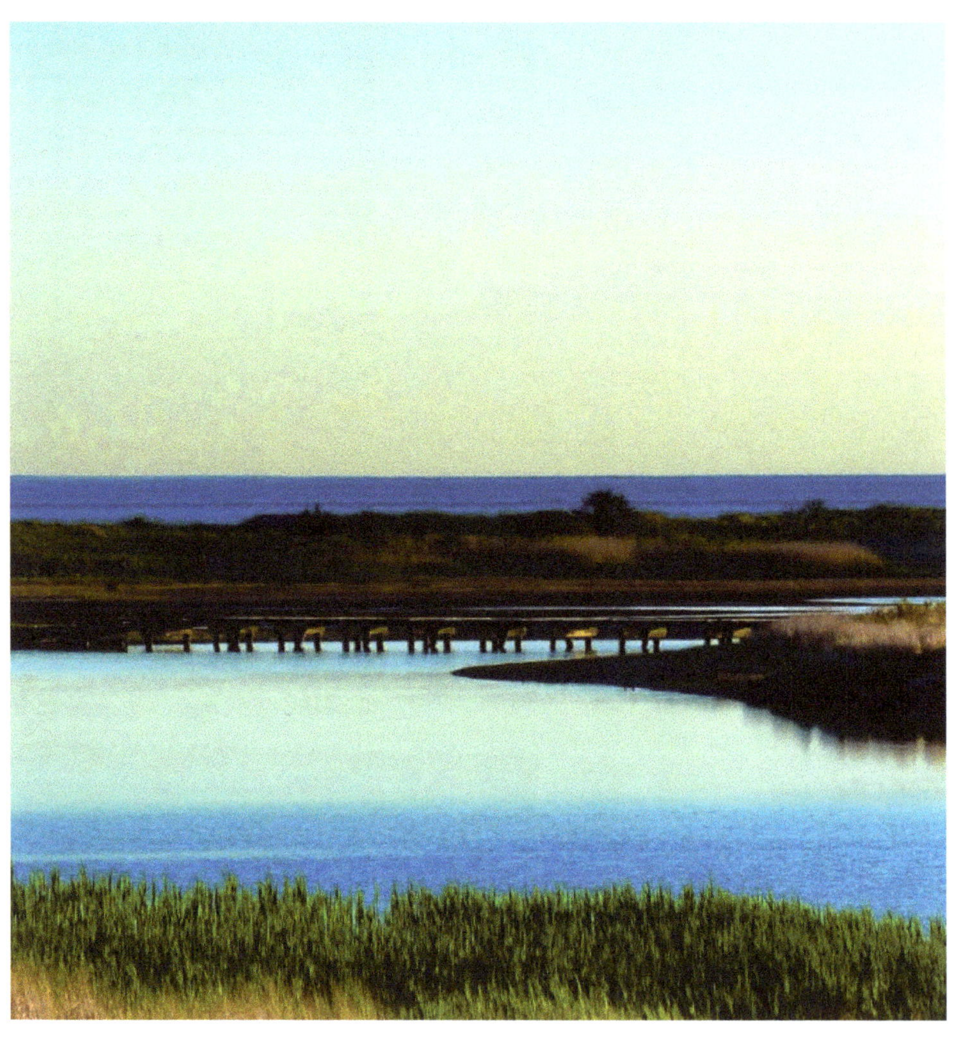

Never settle for less than your dreams,
somewhere, sometime, someday,
somehow you will find them.

—Danielle Steel

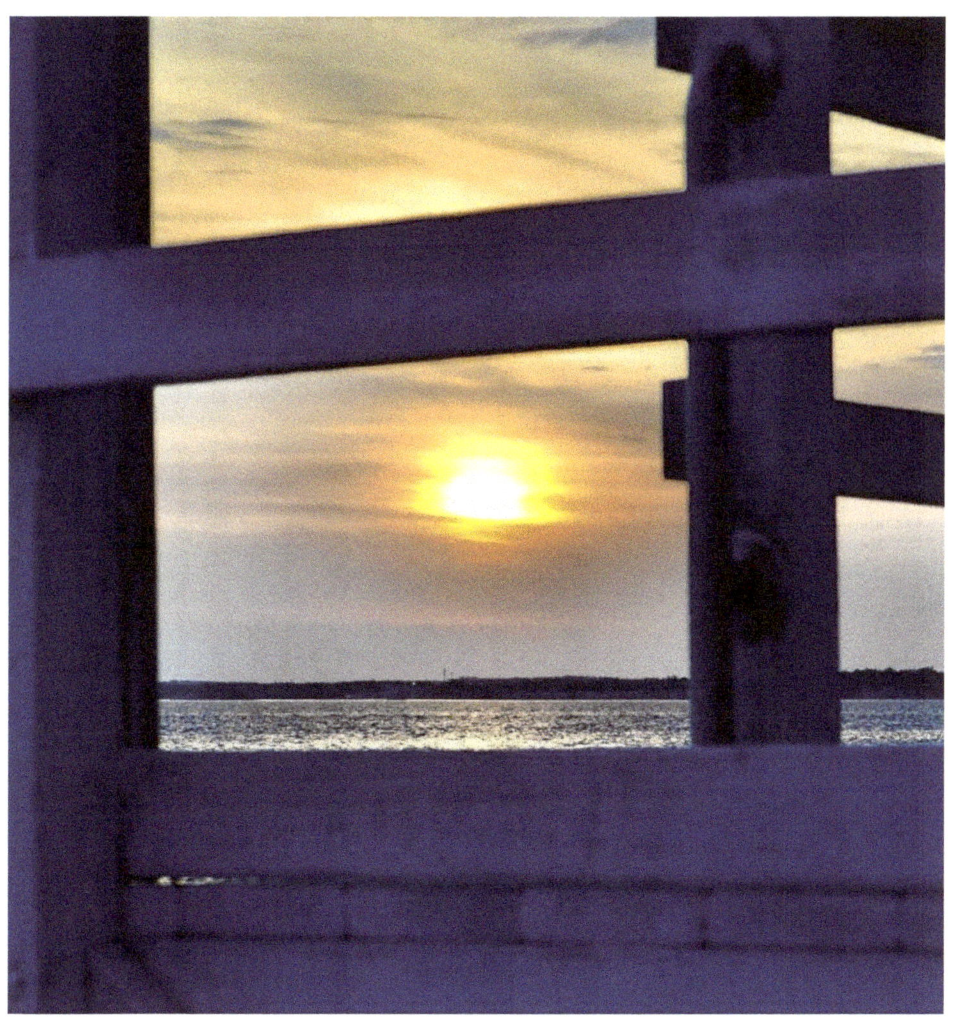

The sun is a daily reminder that we, too,
can rise again from the darkness,
that we, too, can shine our own light.

—S. Anja

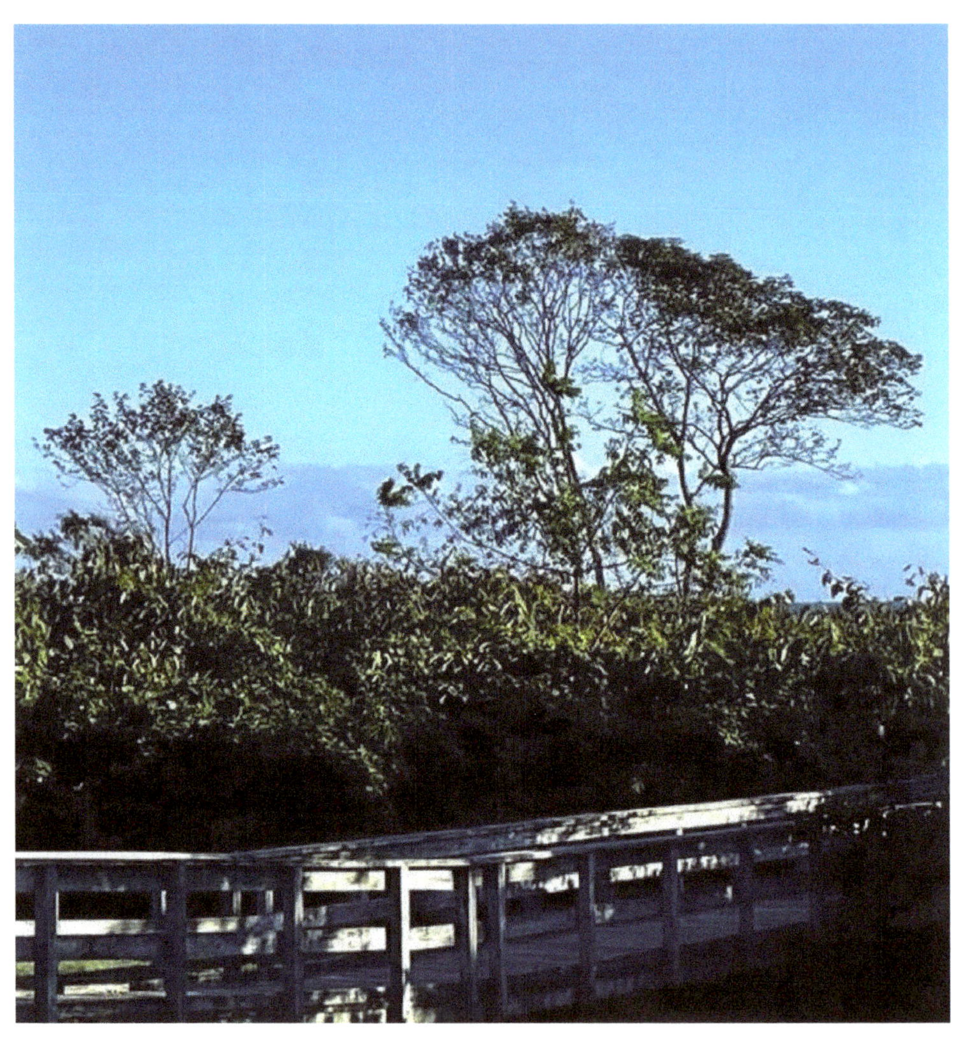

The past is behind, learn from it. The future is ahead, prepare for it. The present is here, live it.

—Thomas S. Monson

CHAPTER 4

Self-Reflecting

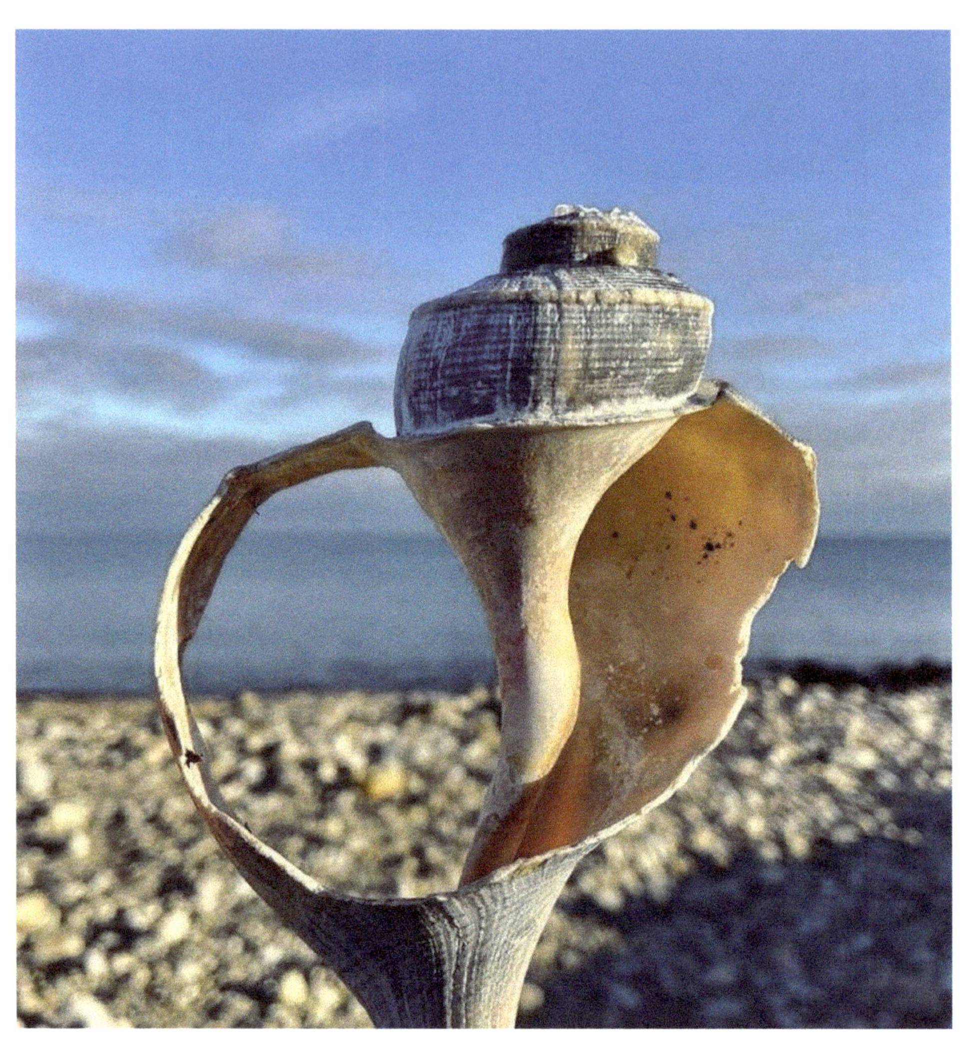

What you think, you become.
What you feel, you attract.
What you imagine, you create.

—Buddha

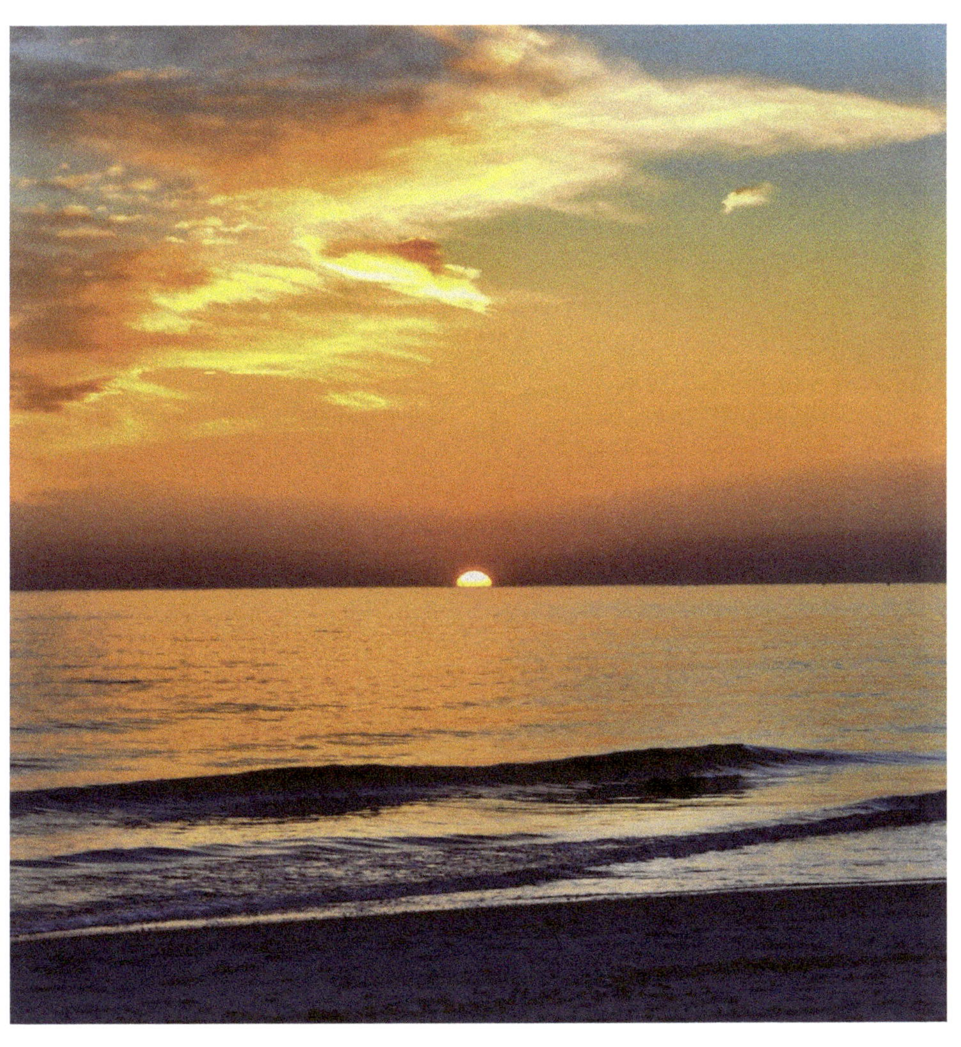

There are two places you need to go to often:
the place that heals you
and the place that inspires you.

—Unknown

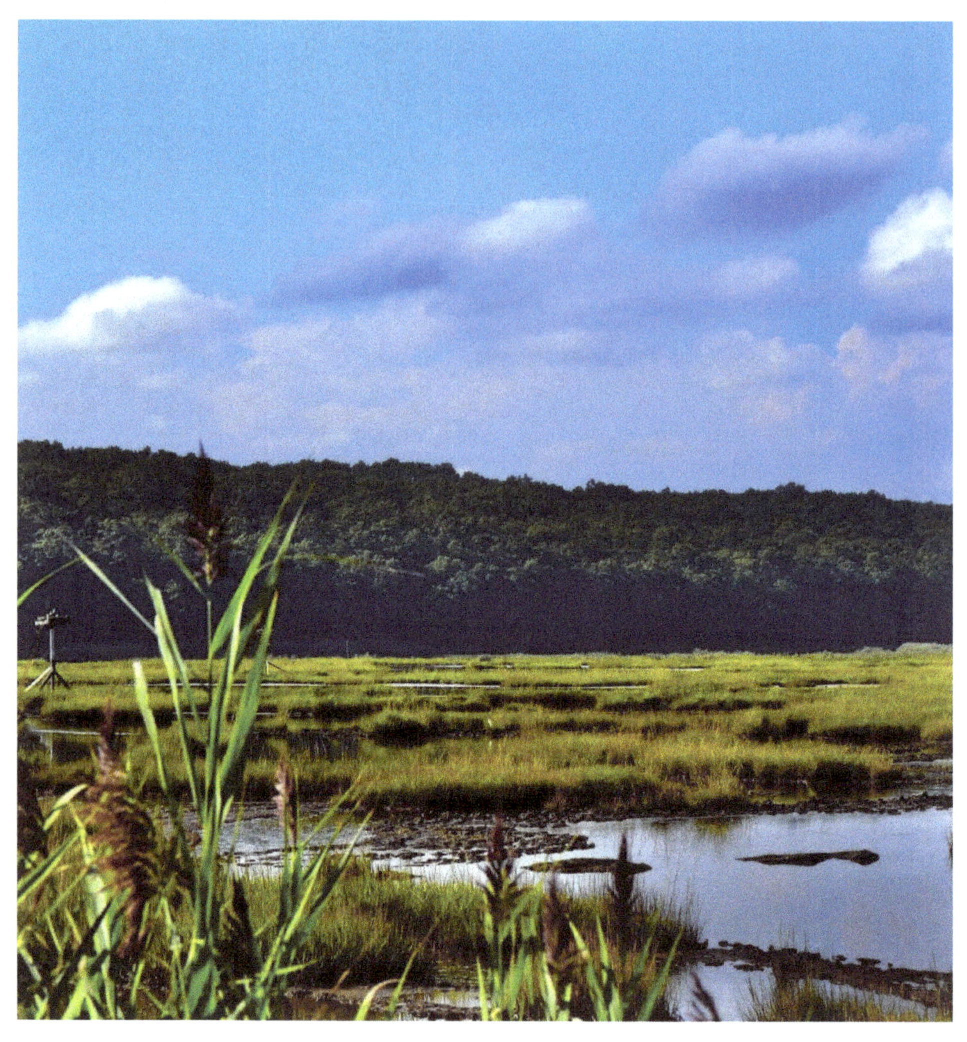

Only what is still can still
the stillness of other things.

—Zhuangzi

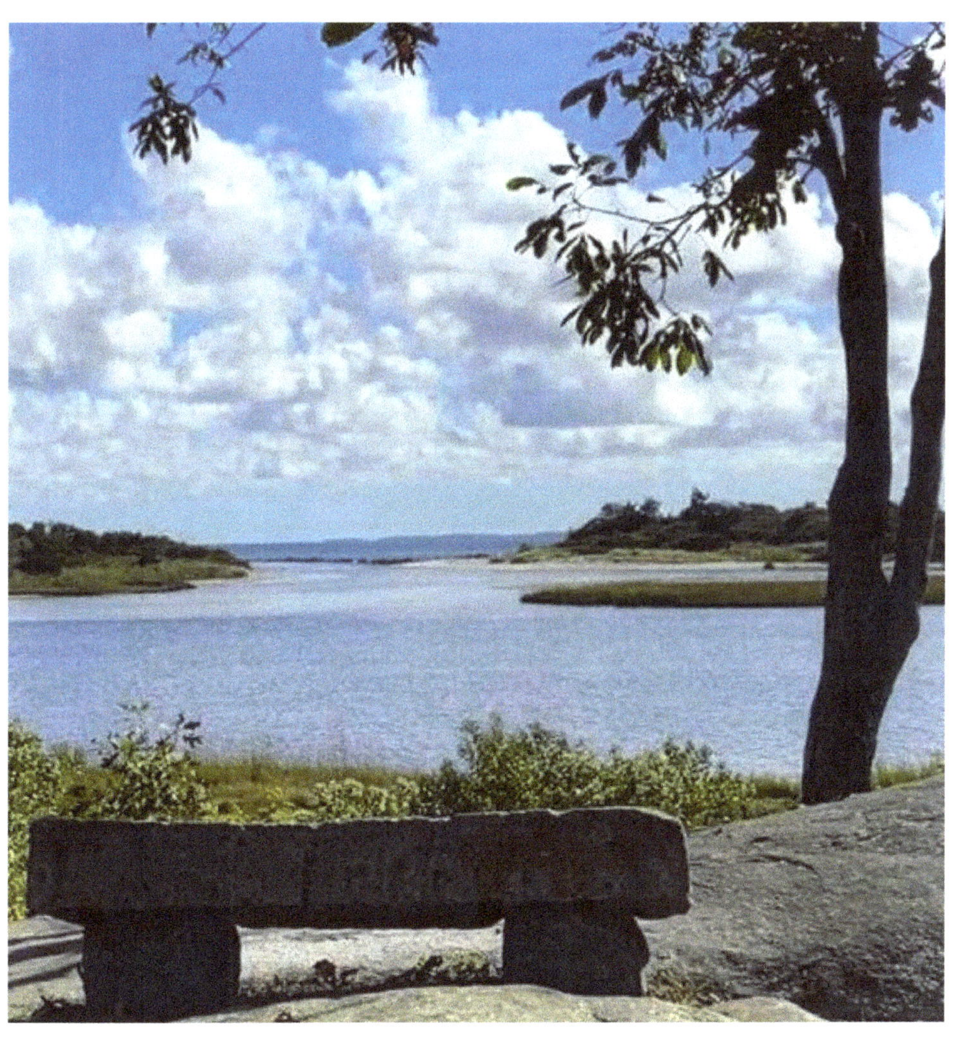

Take time to reflect, relax and just be.

—Unknown

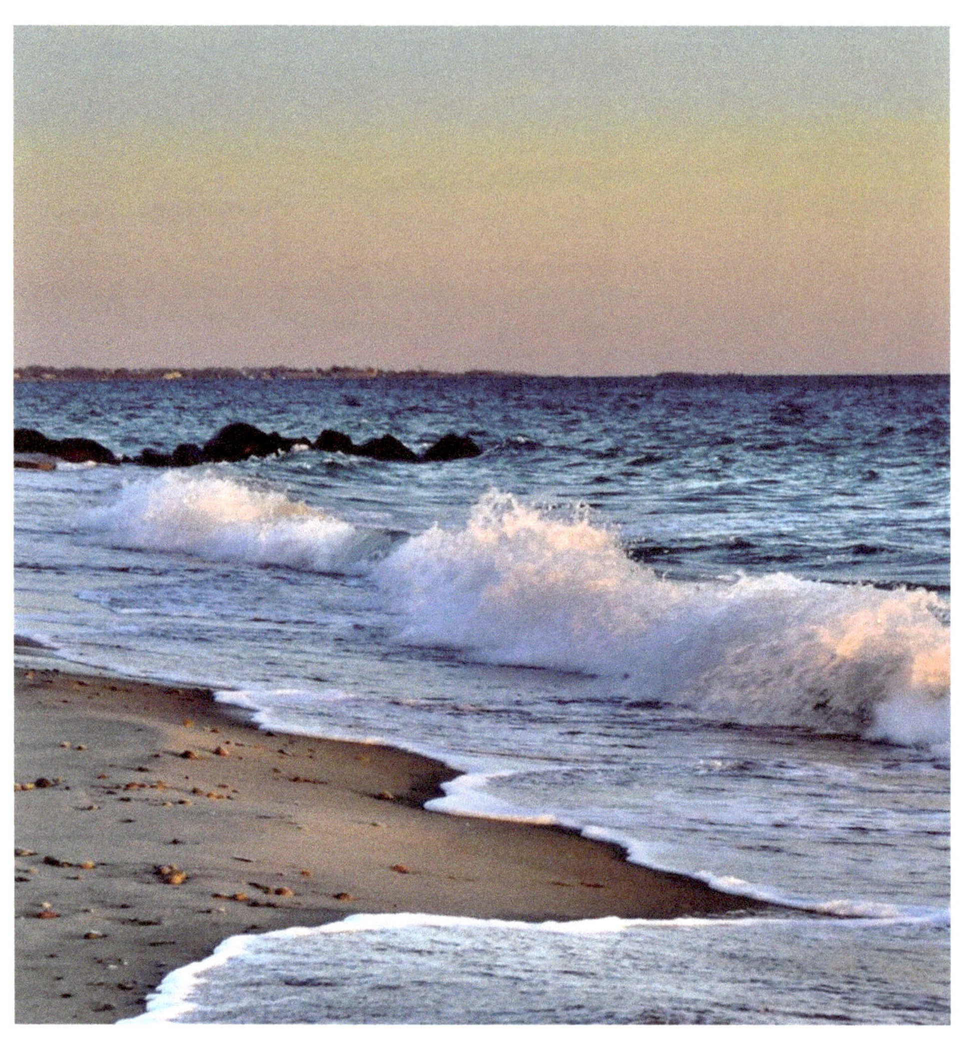

Let the waters settle and you will see
the moon and the stars
mirrored in your own being.

—Rumi

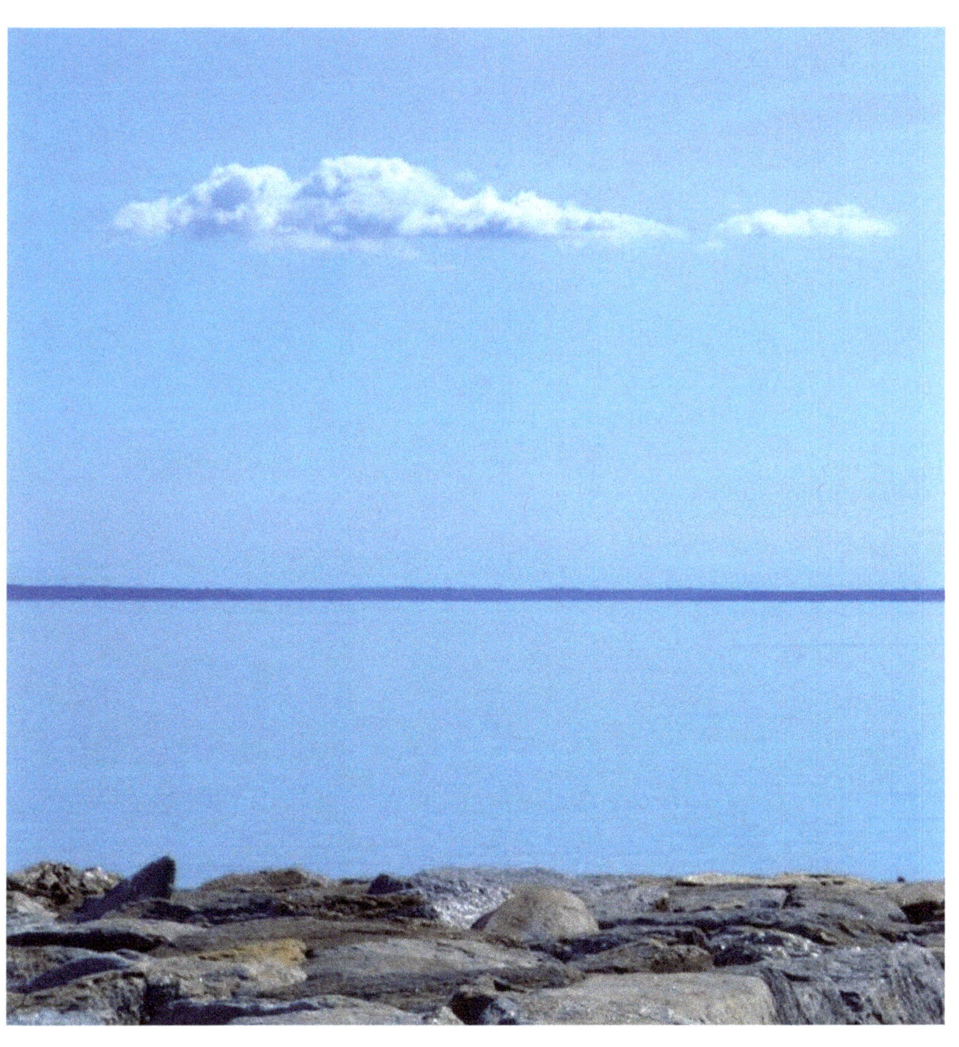

Life is about balance.
Be kind, but don't let people abuse you.
Trust, but don't be deceived.
Be content, but never stop improving yourself.

—Zig Ziglar

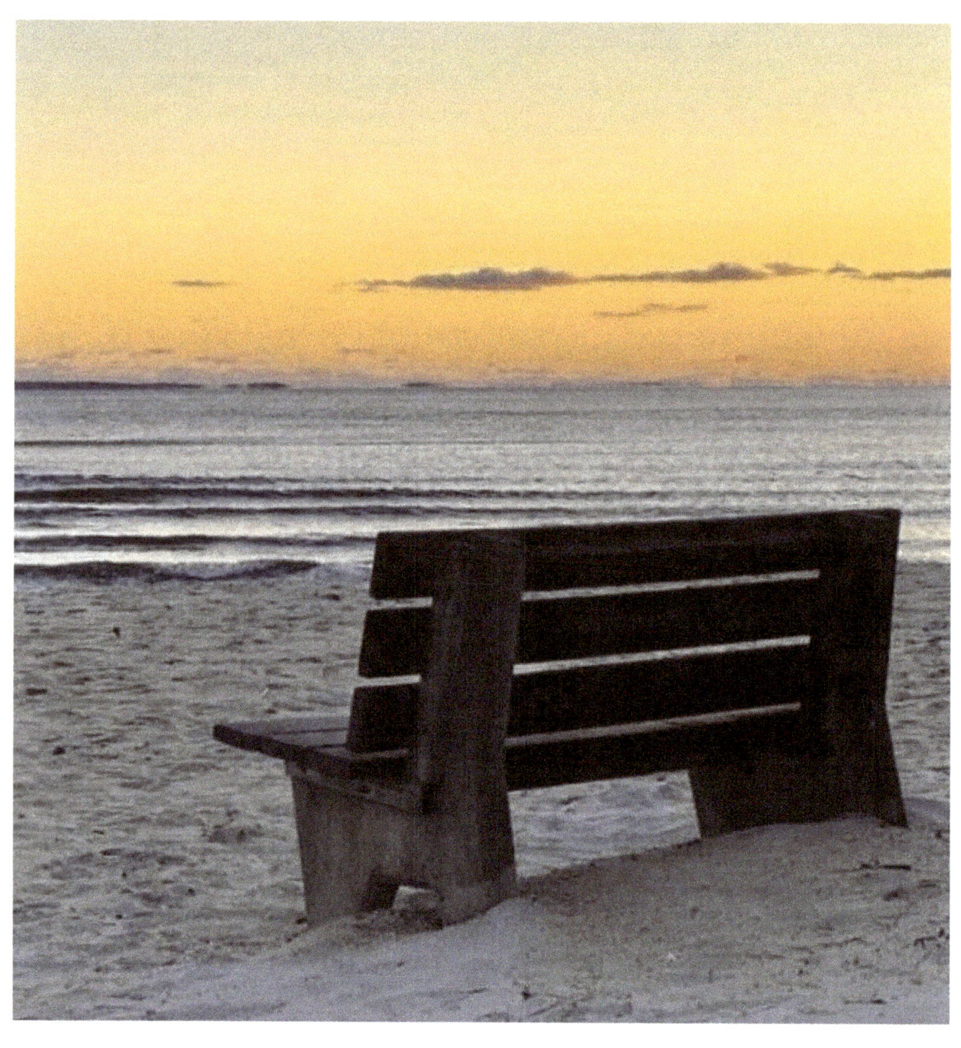

Every morning dedicate a few moments
to breathe in who you truly are.

—Roxana Jones

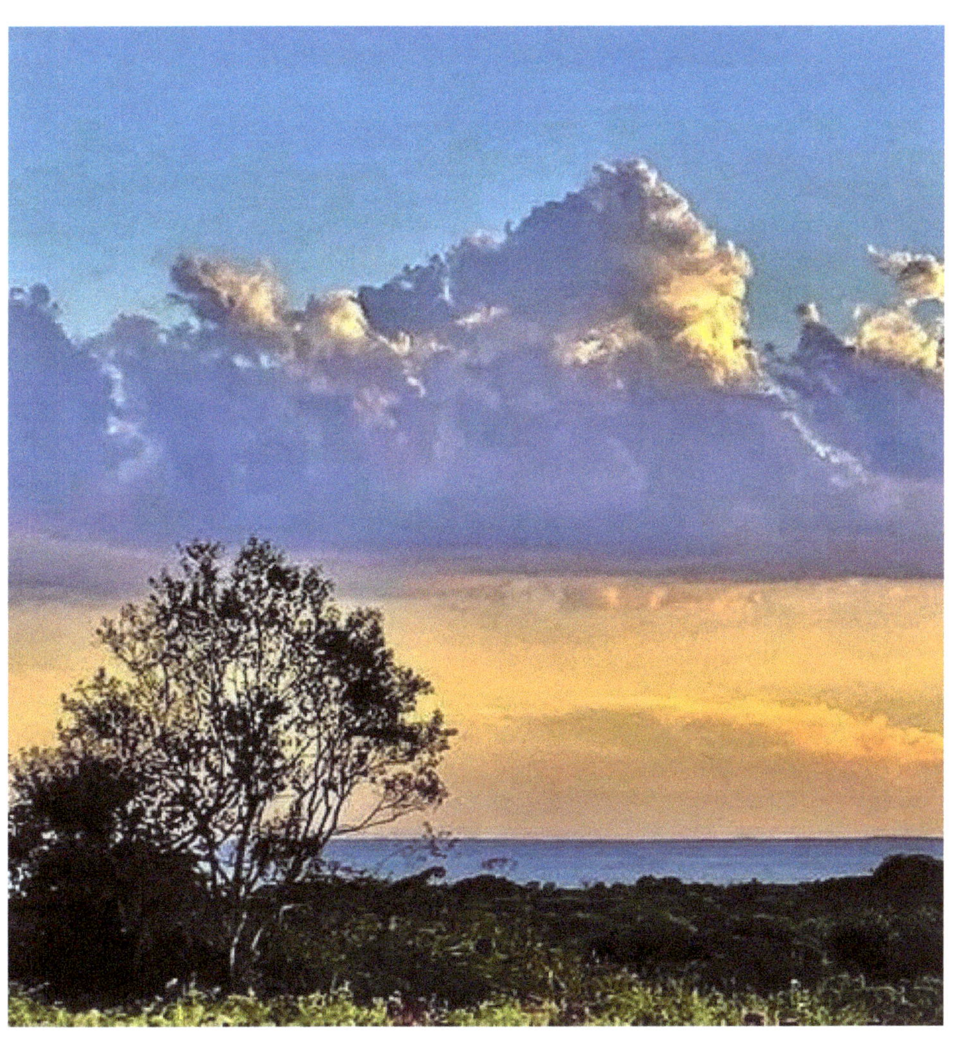

I've looked at clouds from both sides now.
From up and down and still somehow.
It's cloud's illusions I recall.
I really don't know clouds at all.

—Judy Collins

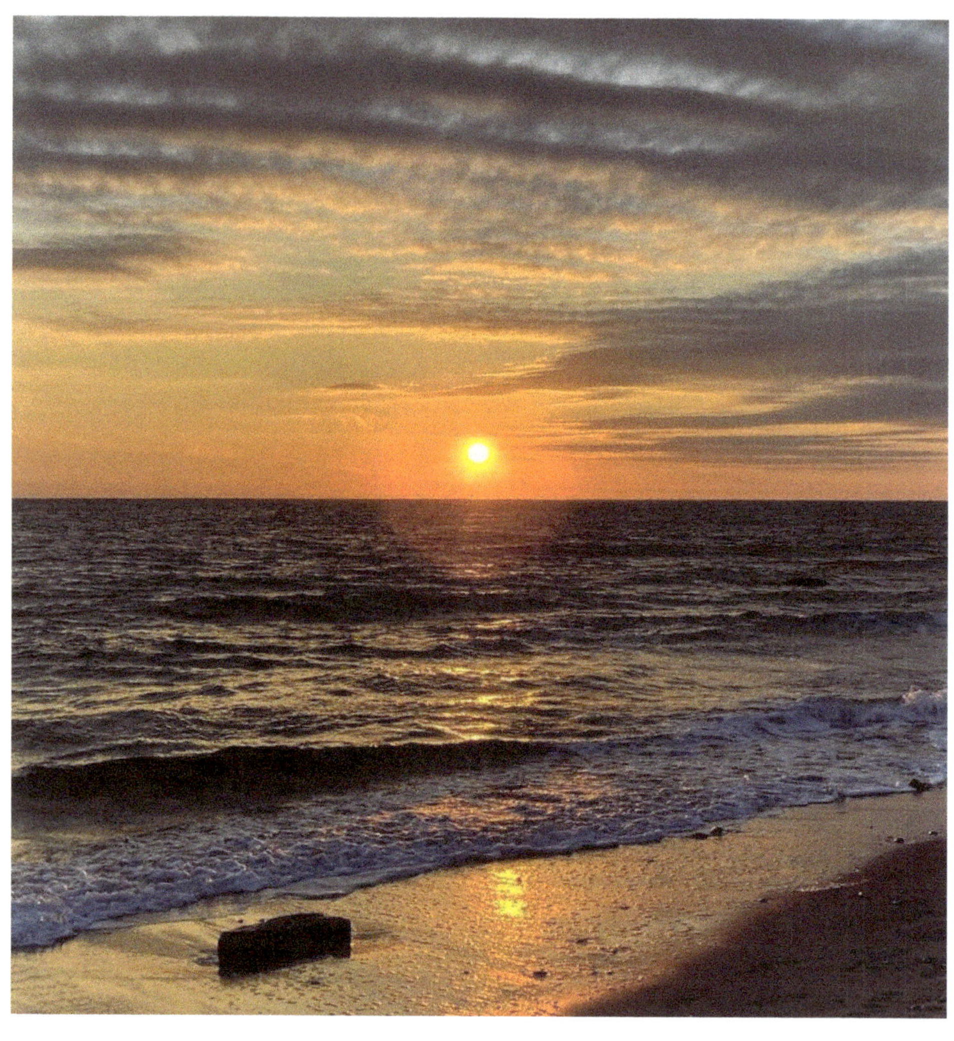

I went down to the sea again today,
And tried to make my worries go away.
I lay down on the sand and closed my eyes,
And listened to the sea sing lullabies.

—Sandy Coleman

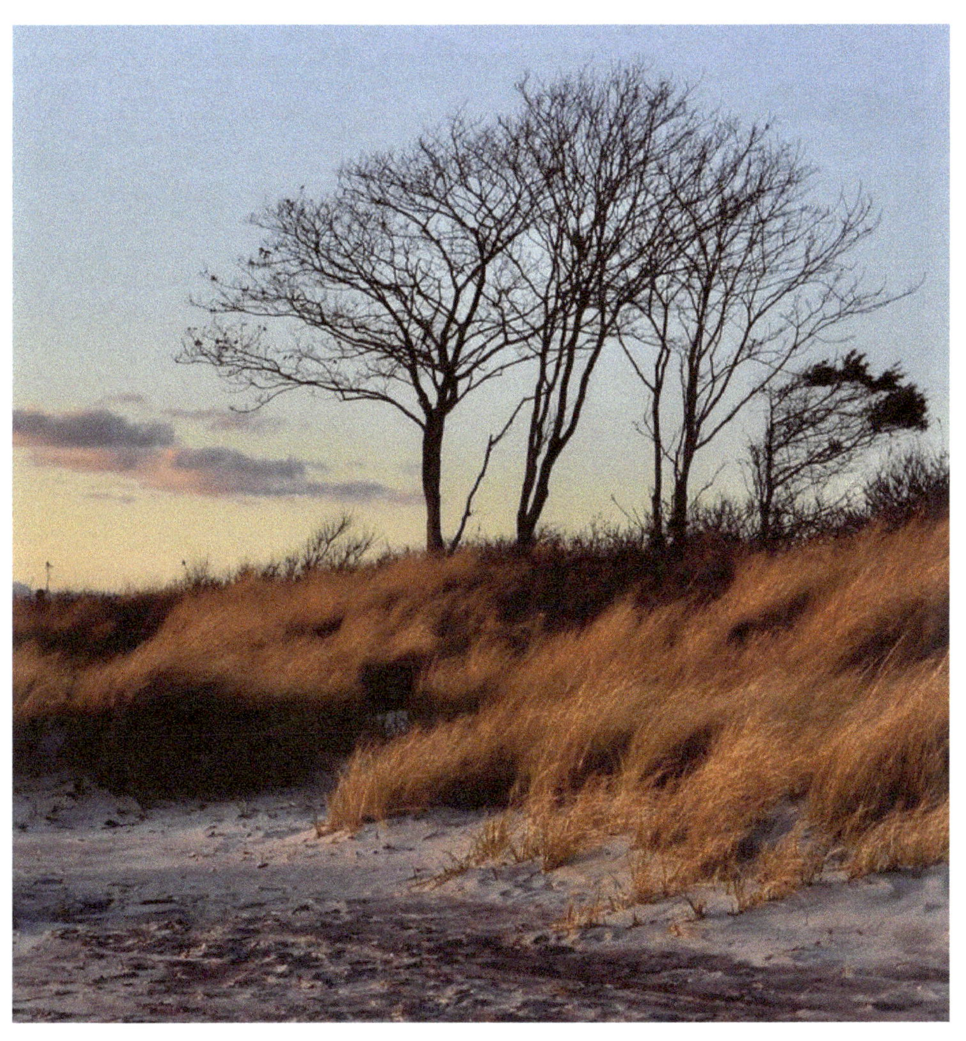

There's never been a better time
to let the leaves of mediocrity
fall from your tree of life.

—David Ault

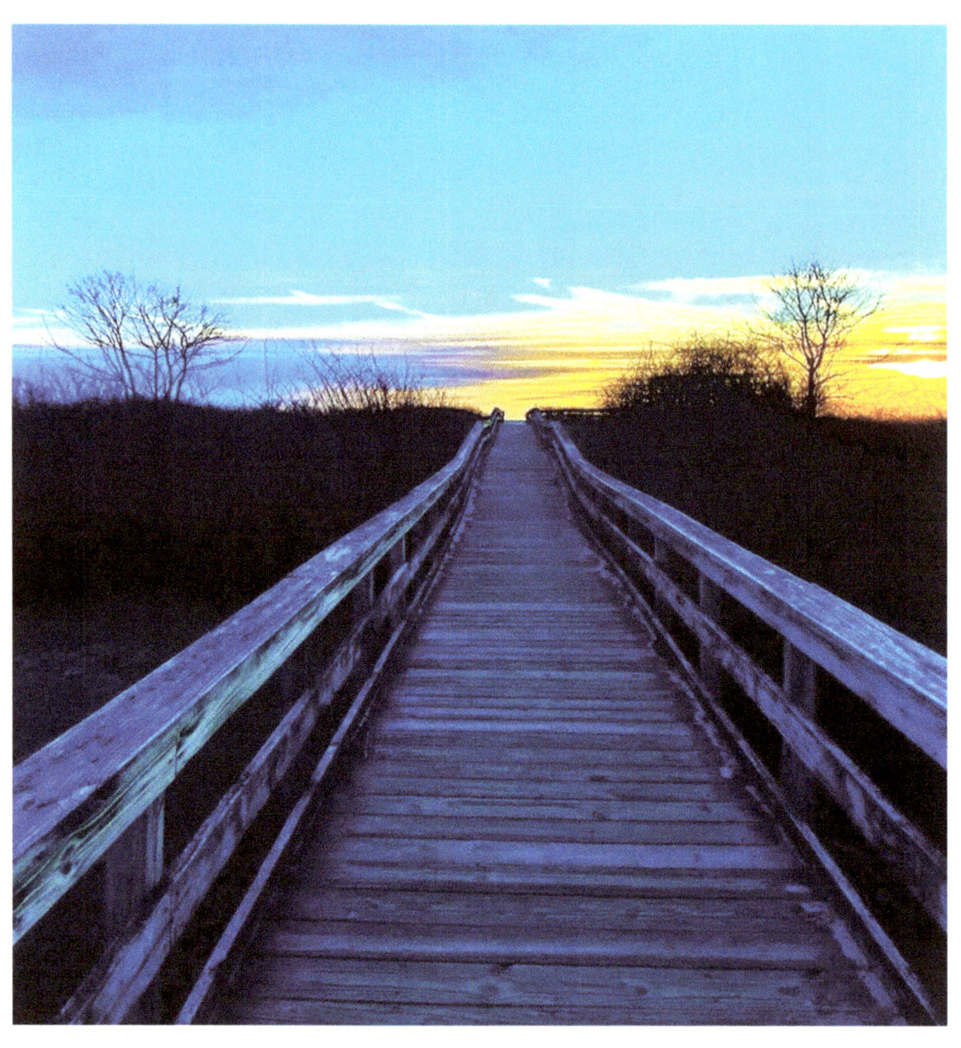

In every walk with nature
one receives far more than he seeks.

—John Muir

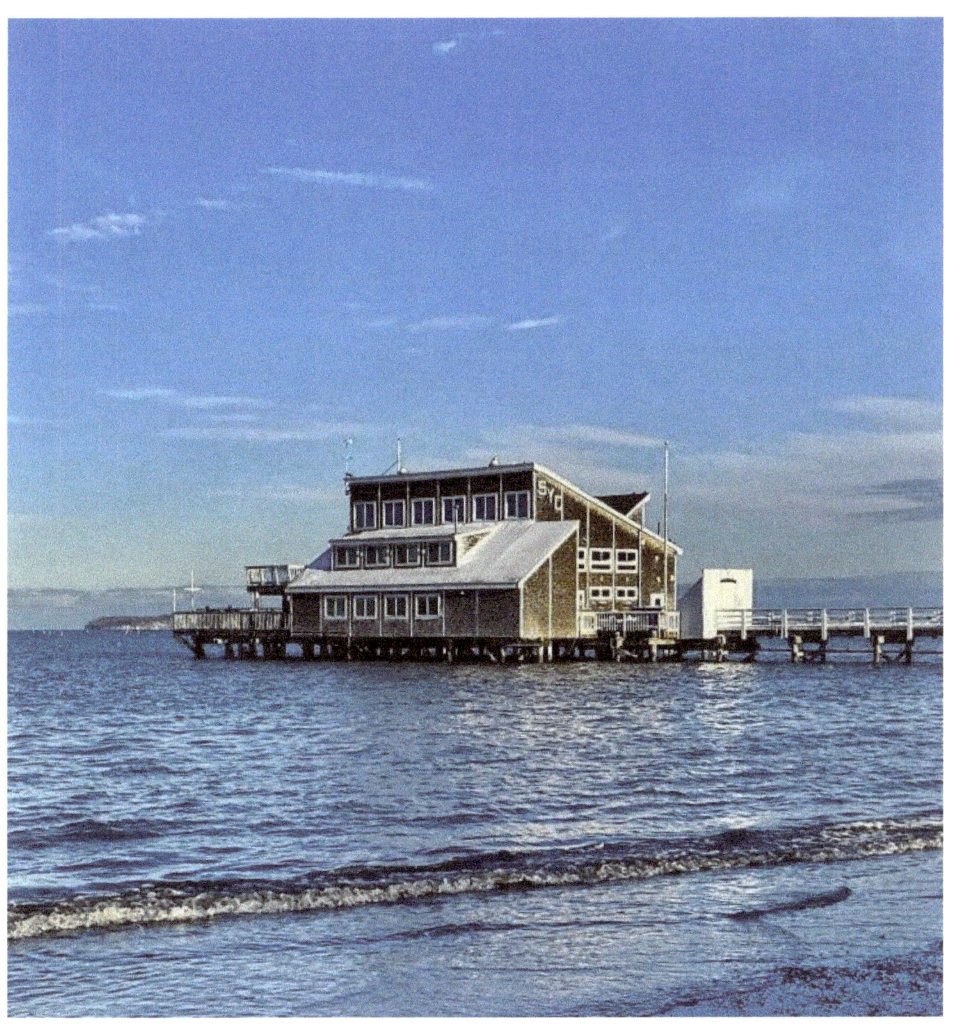

The secret of change is to focus all of your energy not on fighting the old, but on building the new.

—Socrates

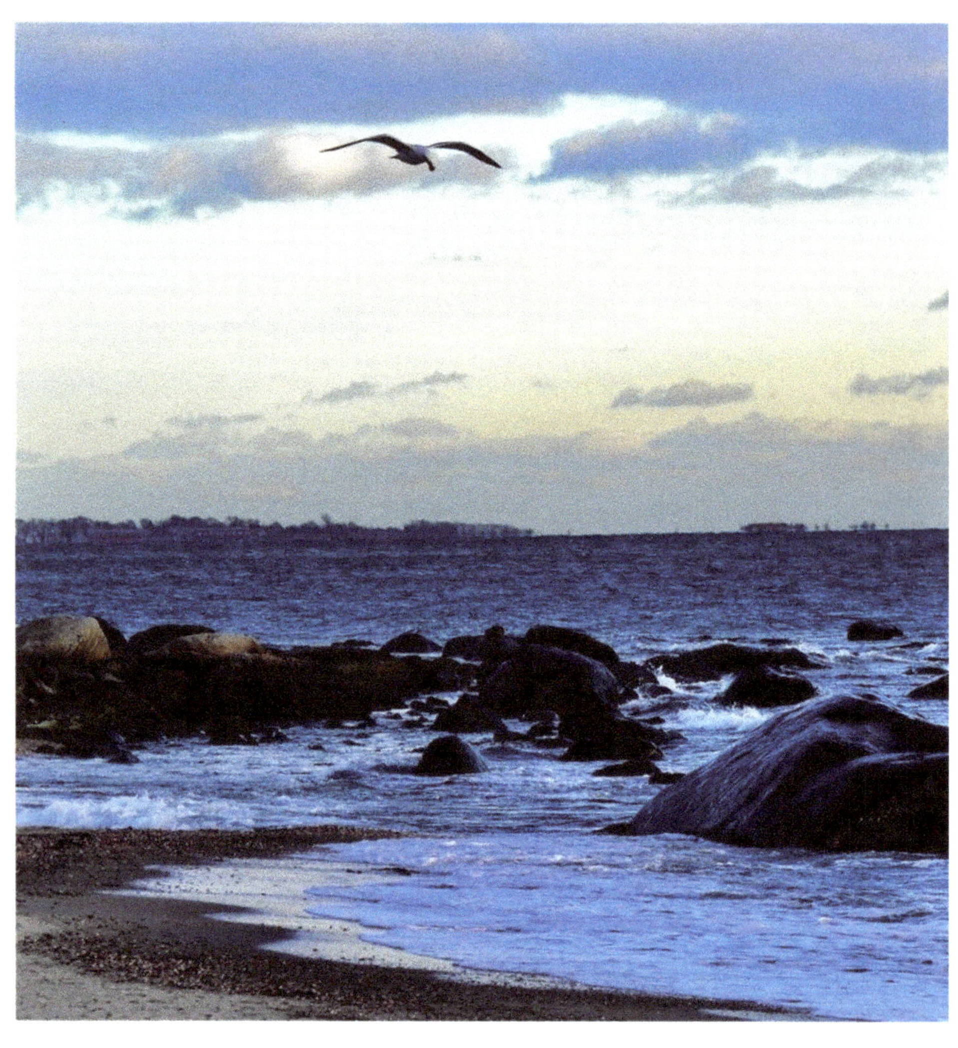

Sometimes I want to ask God why He allows poverty, famine and injustice in the world when he could do something about it, but I'm afraid he might ask me the SAME QUESTION.

—Brandon Hatmaker

CHAPTER 5

Stepping Out of Your Comfort Zone

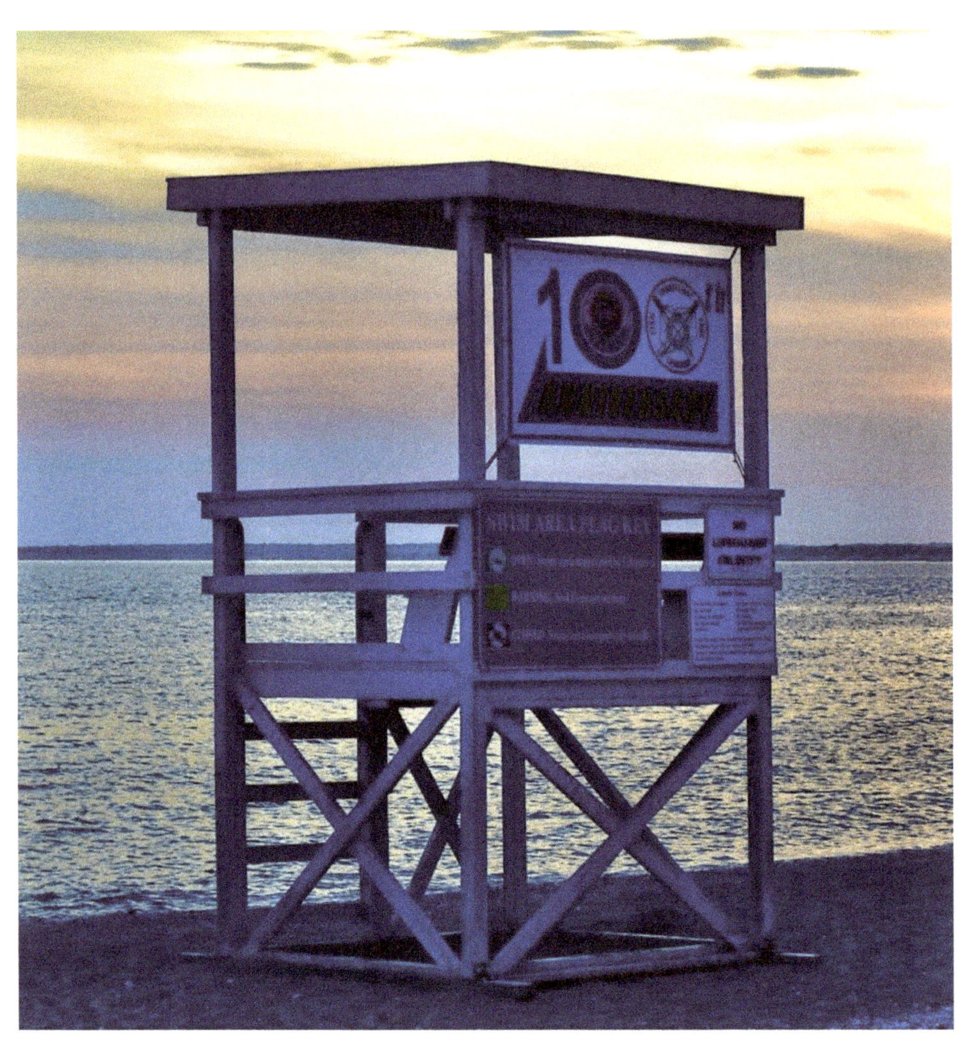

There is no lifeguard on duty.
We each swim at our risk during this journey.

—Lisa Fantino

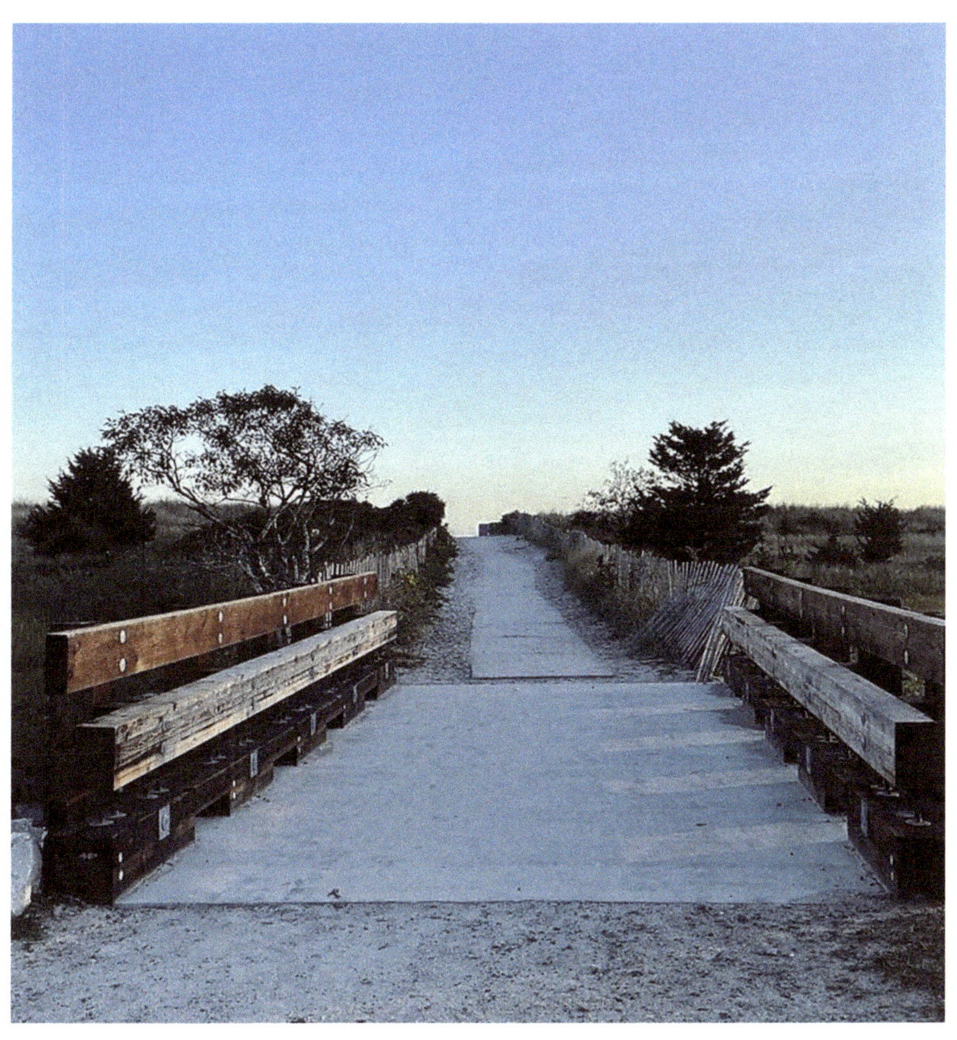

You can't get to courage without walking through vulnerability.

—Brené Brown

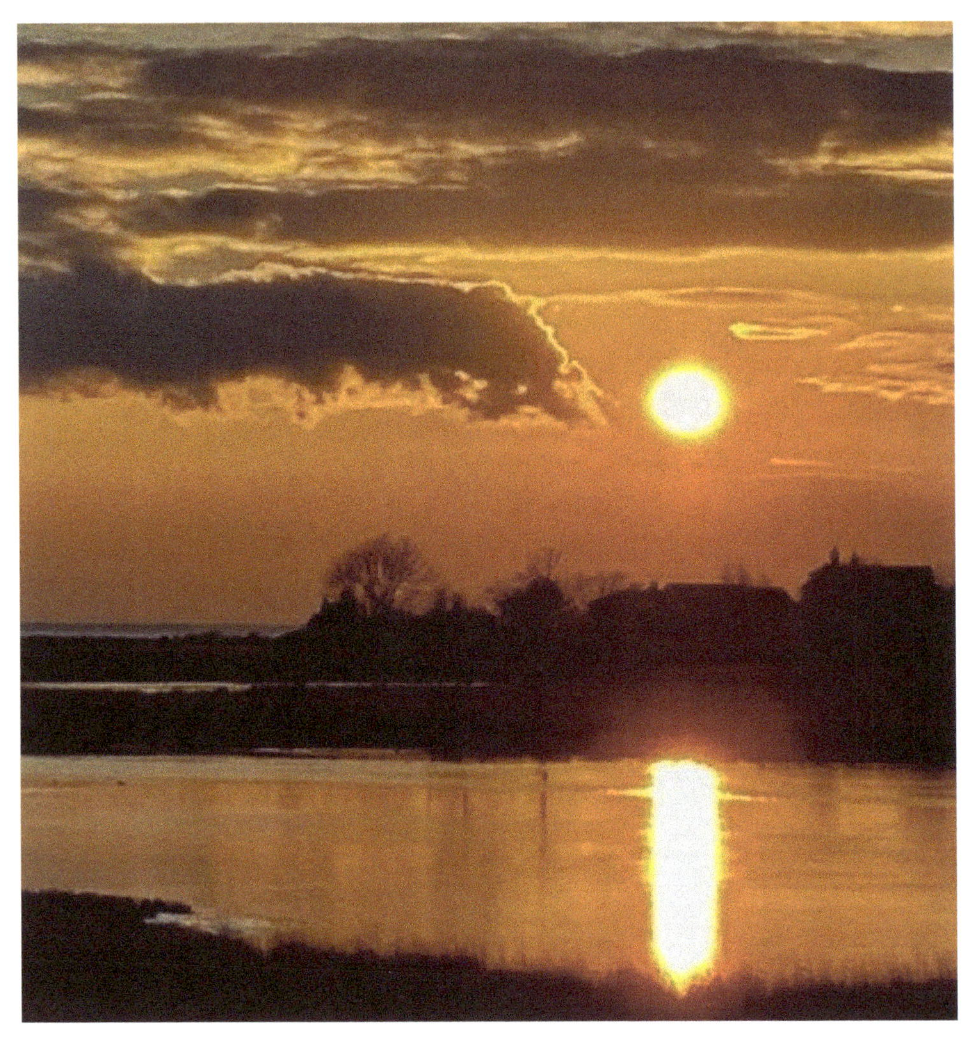

If you look at the people in your circle
and don't get inspired,
then you don't have a circle.
You have a cage.

—Nipsey Hussle

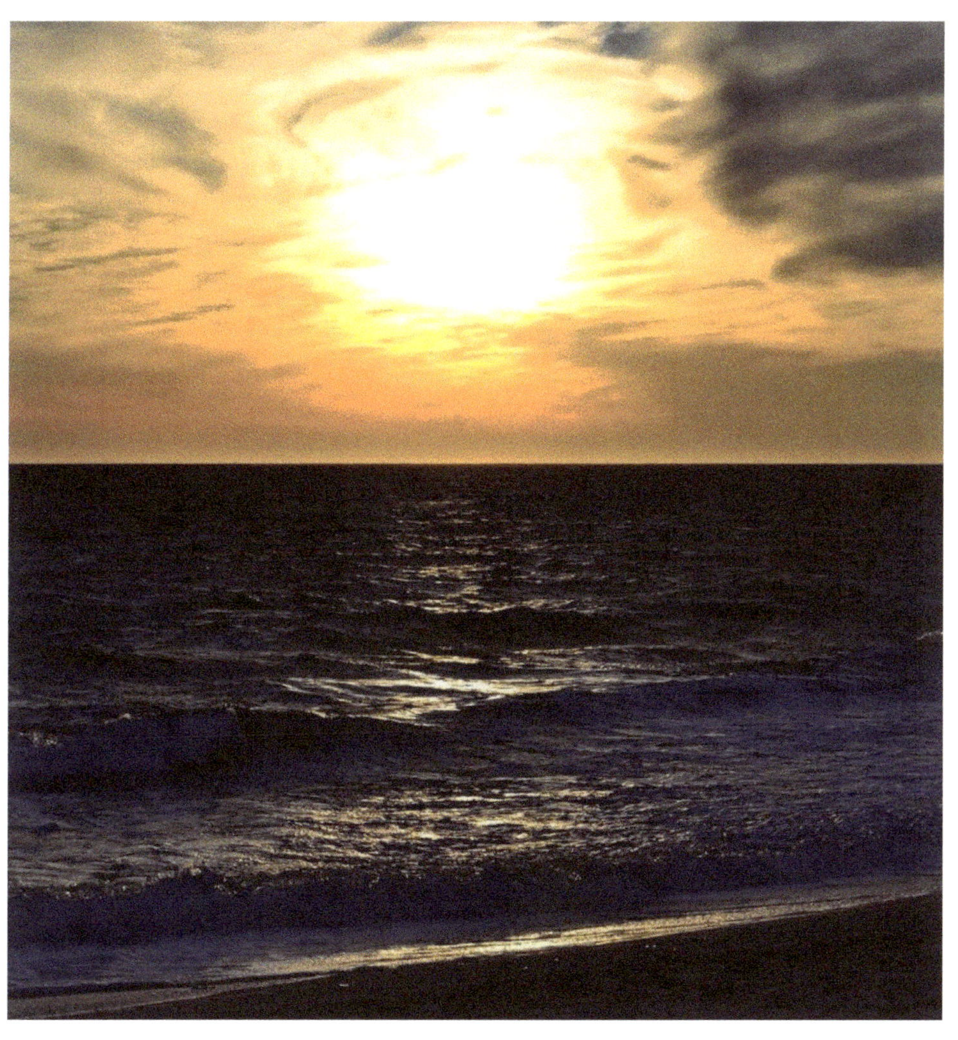

For there is always light,
if only we're brave enough to see it.
If only we're brave enough to be it.

—Amanda Gorman

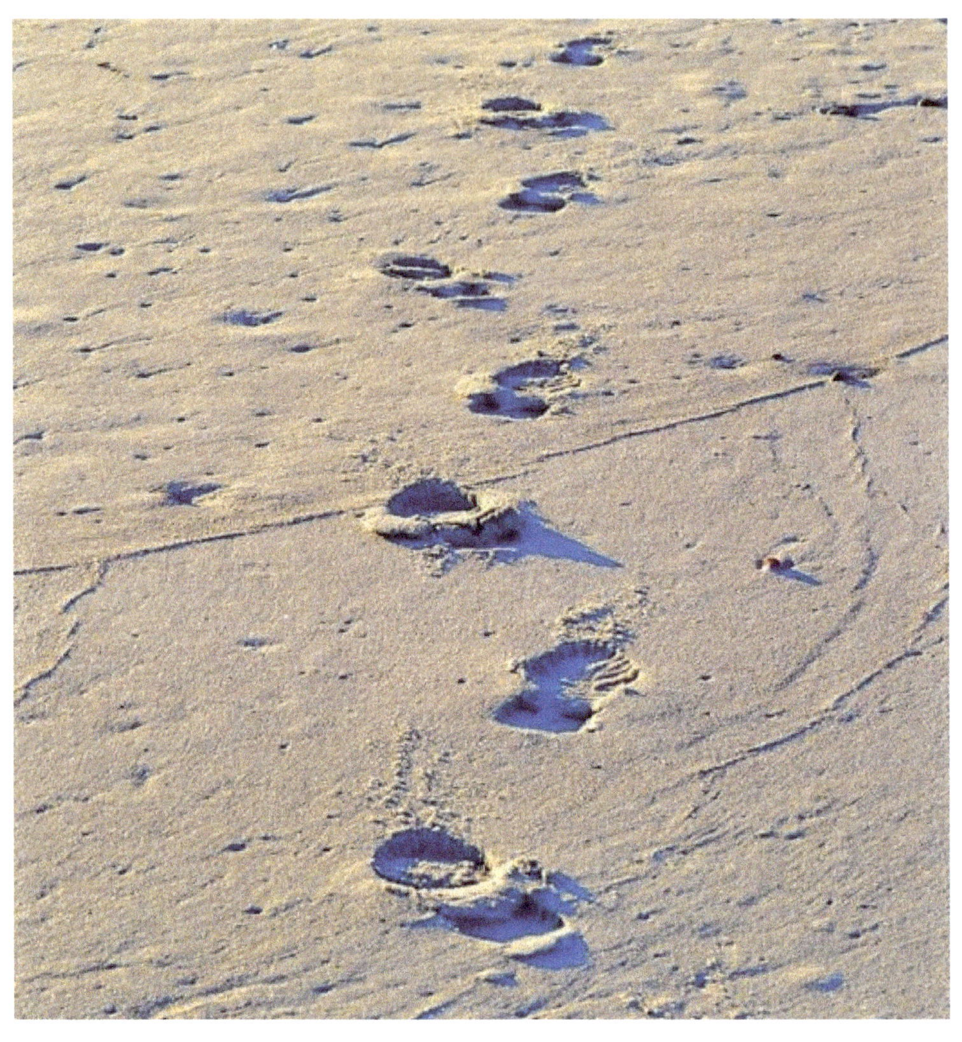

You can't leave footprints in the sands of time while sitting down.

—Nelson Rockefeller

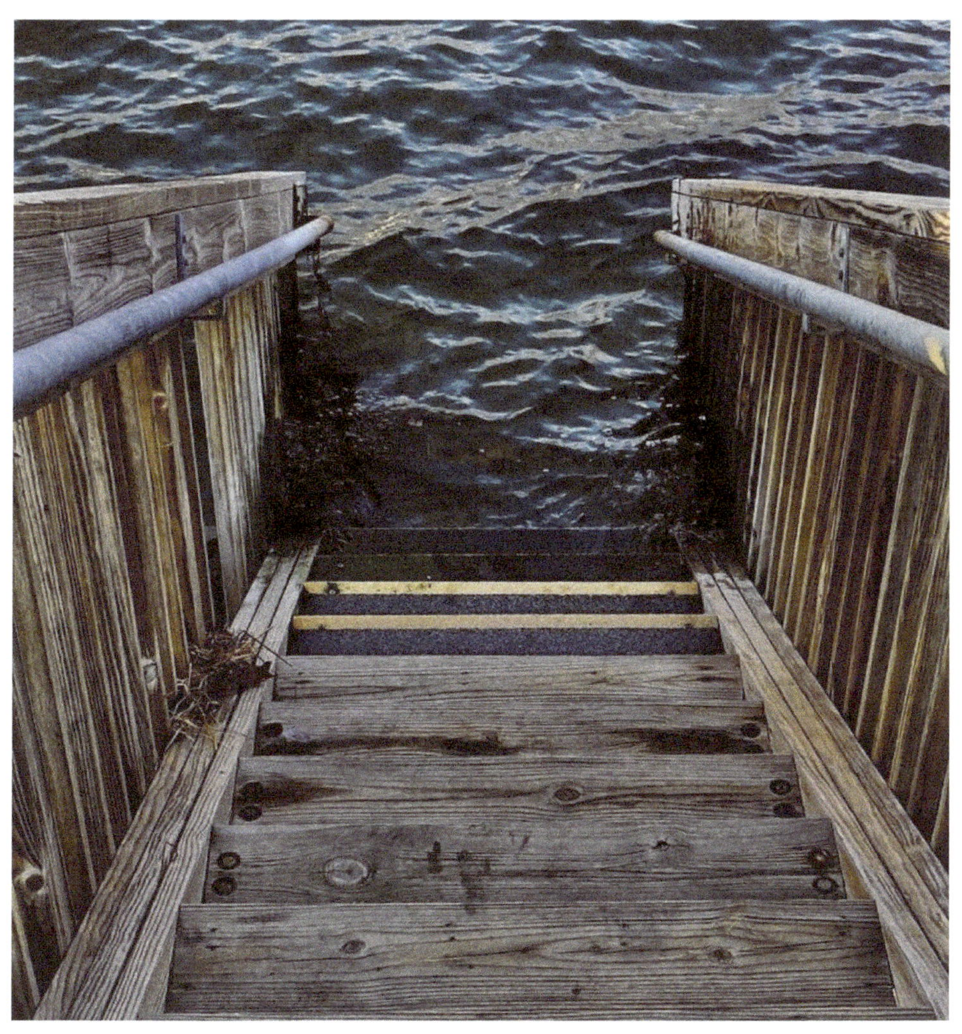

The miracle is not to walk on water.
The miracle is to walk on earth.

—Linjl Yixuan

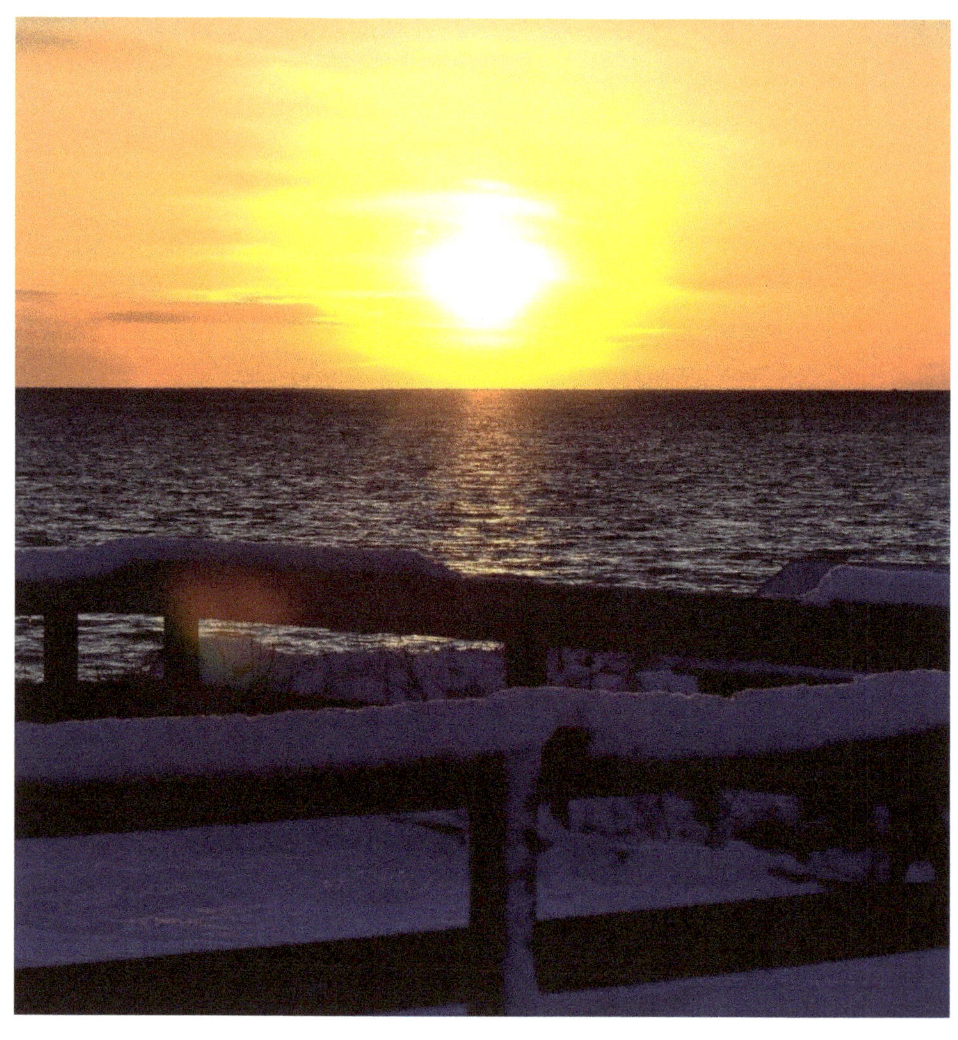

Change is inevitable.
Growth is optional.

—John C. Maxwell

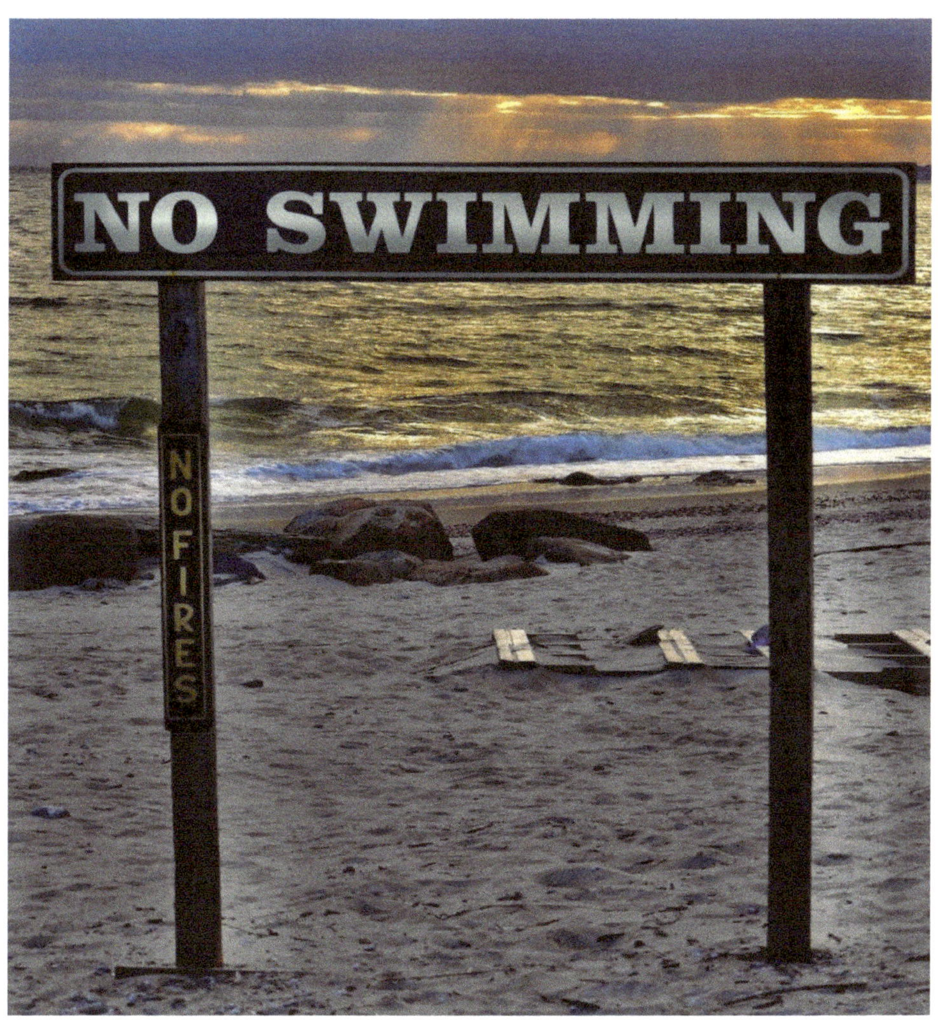

You either walk inside your story and own it,
or you stand outside your story
and hustle for your worthiness.

—Brené Brown

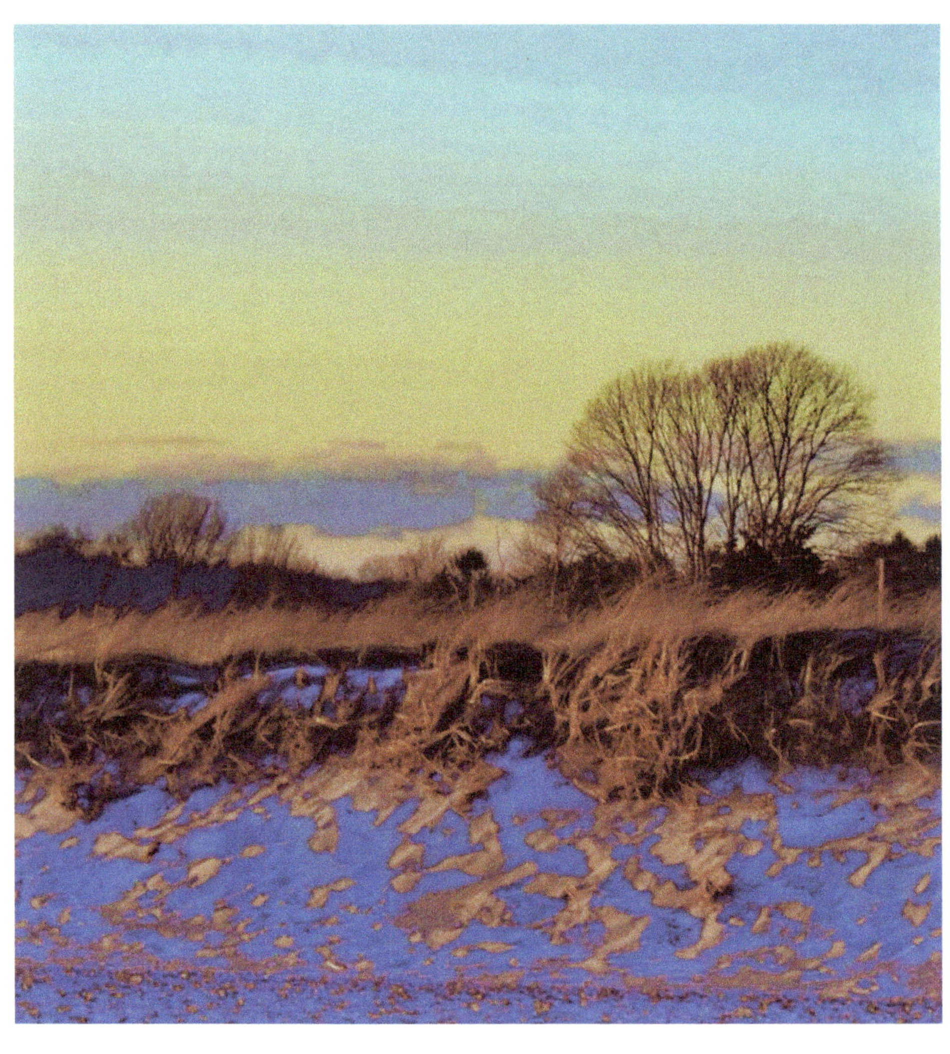

Accept your past without regret,
handle your presence with confidence
and face your future without fear.

—Shruti Gaja

CHAPTER 6

Finding Direction and Purpose

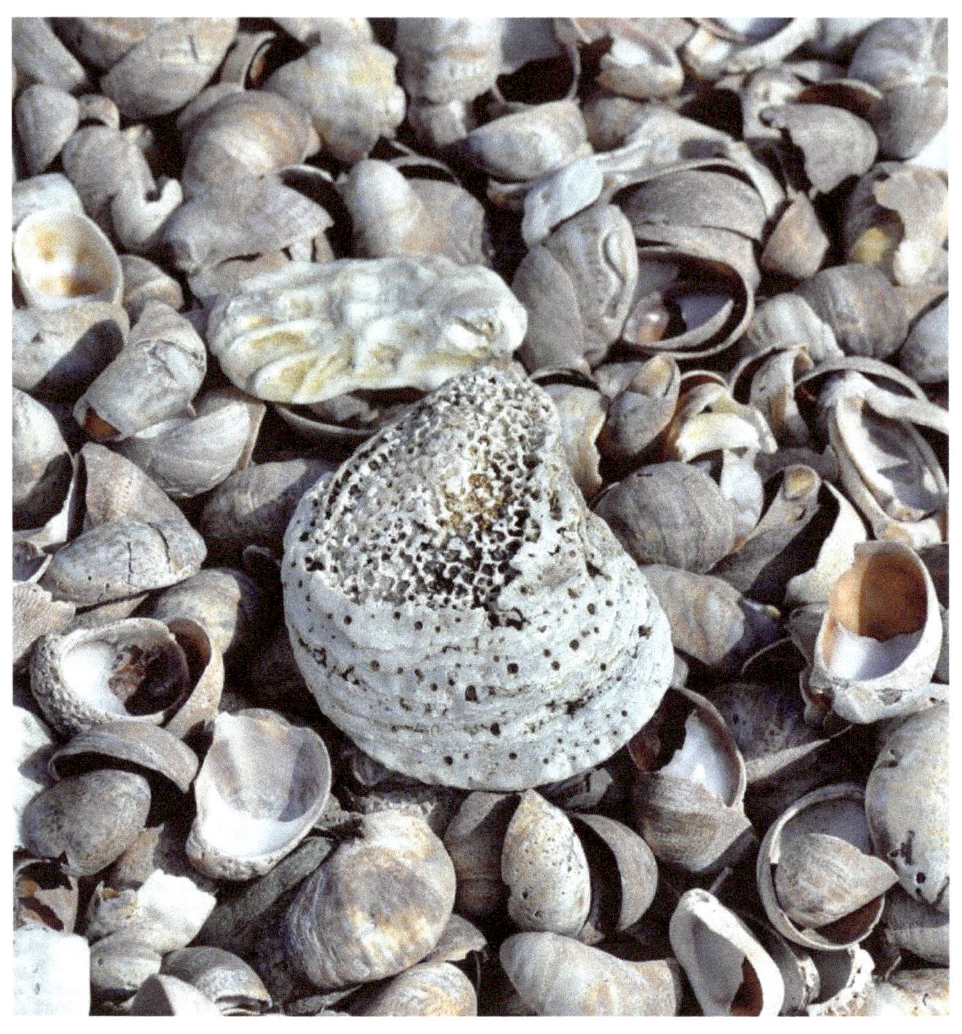

We are like seashells upon the beach,
beautiful and unique,
each with a story of its own to tell.

—Unknown

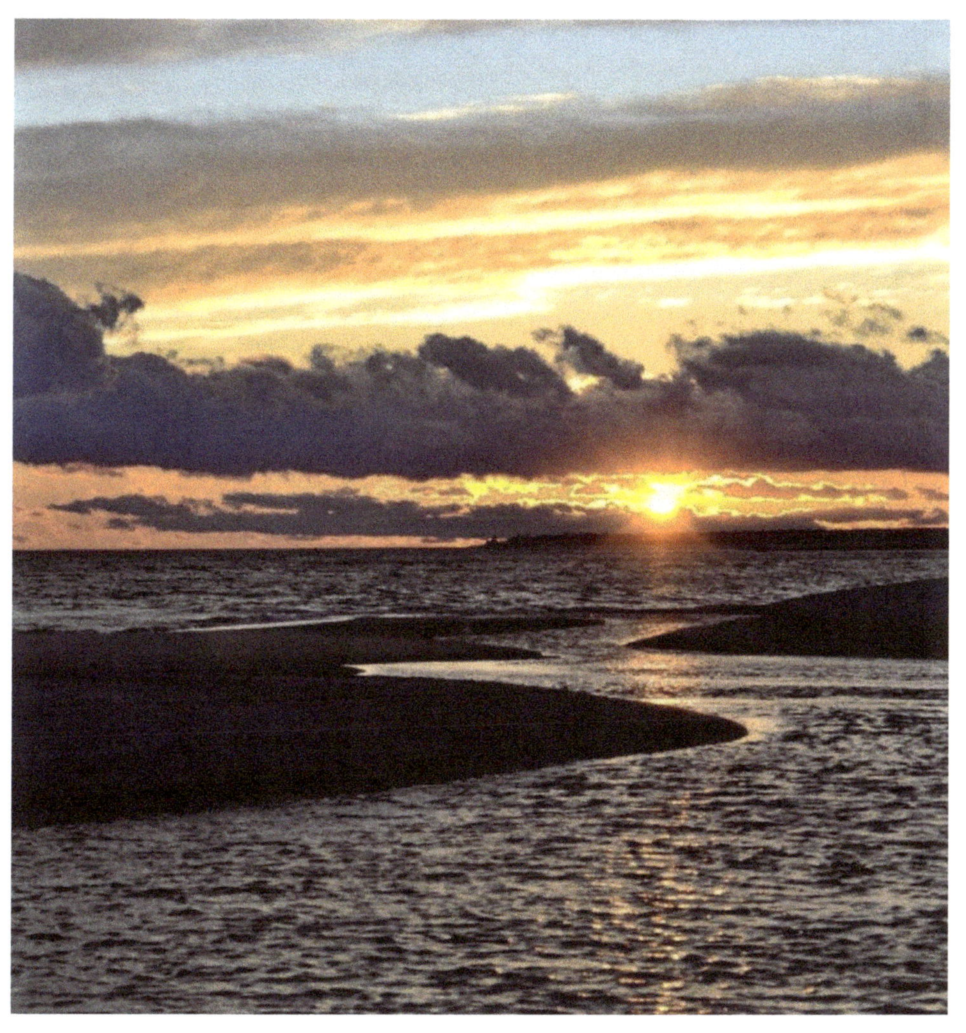

Follow your passion
and good things will happen.

—Dr. Miguel Cardona

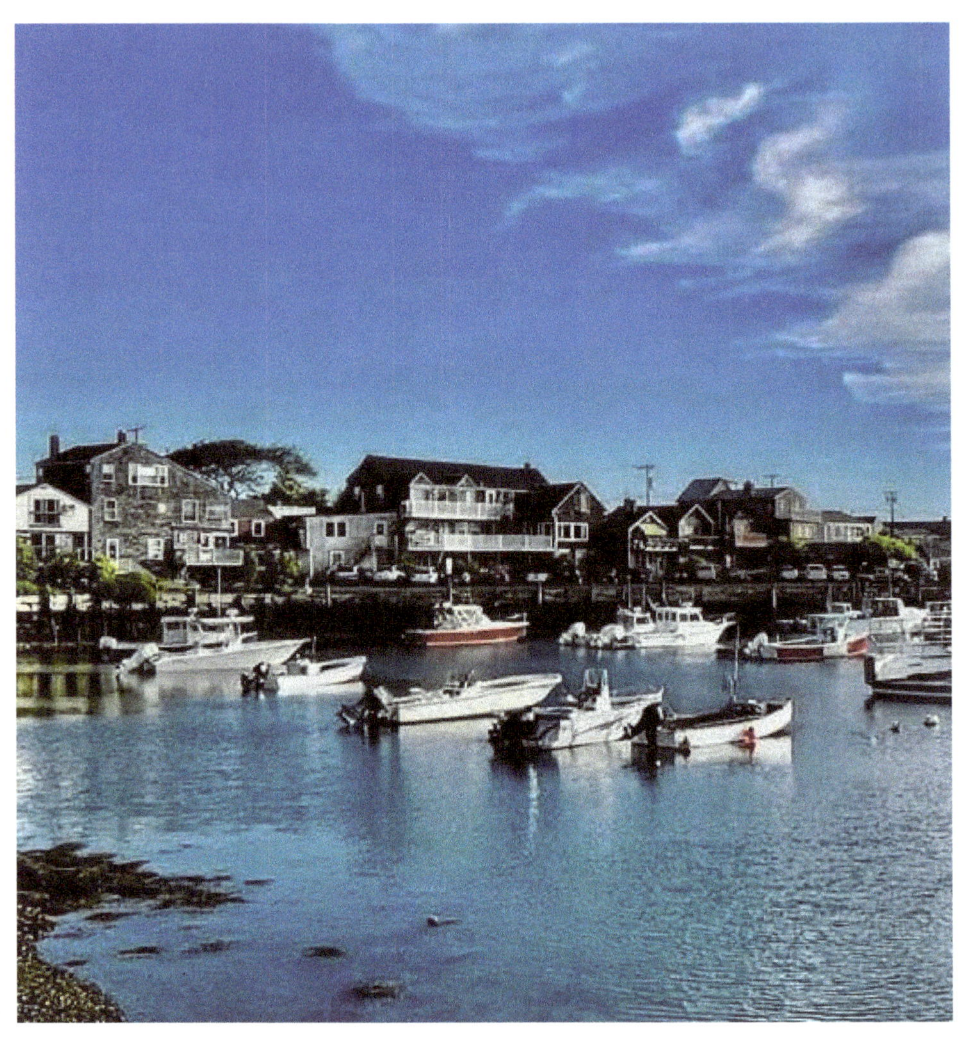

Life without a defined purpose
is similar to a boat without a crew
in the middle of the ocean.

—Debasish Mridha, M.D.

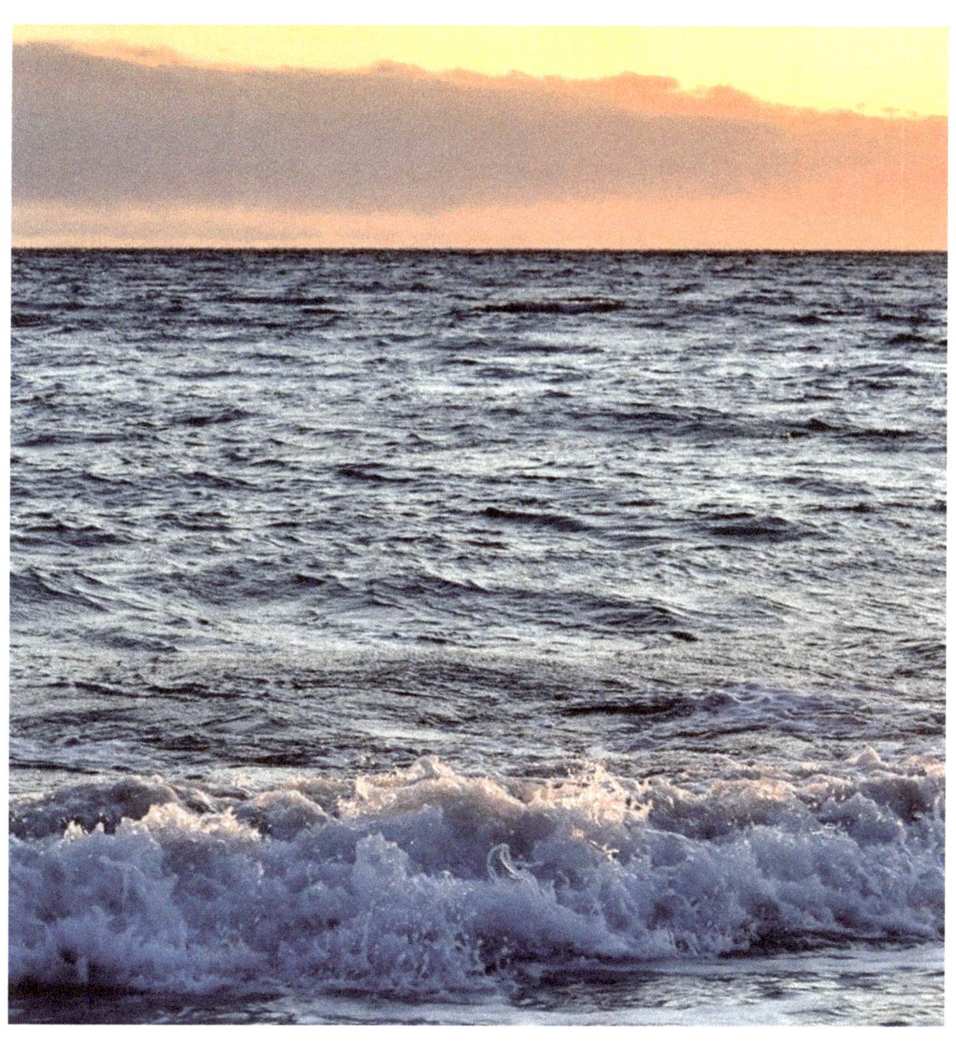

Forgive others,
not because they deserve forgiveness,
but because you deserve peace.

—Jonathan Lockwood Huie

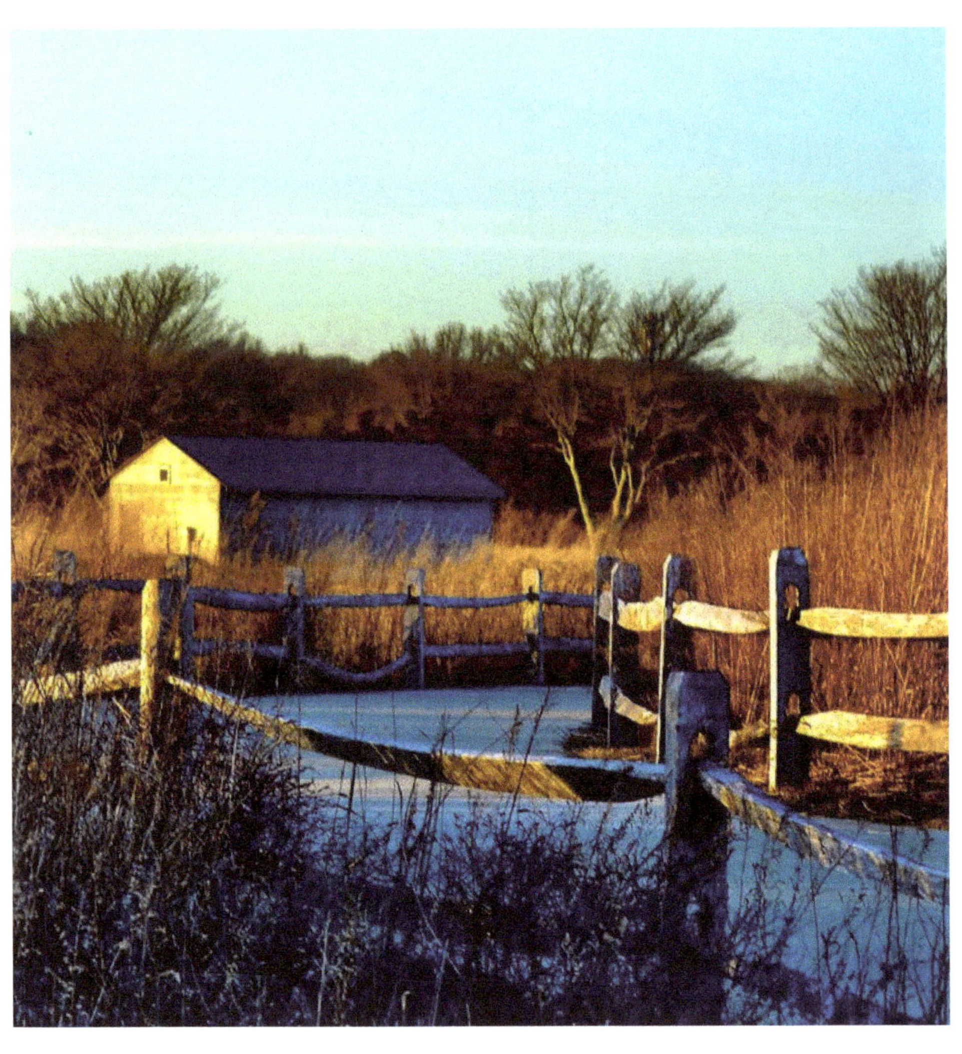

Sometimes you find yourself
in the middle of nowhere;
and sometimes, in the middle of nowhere,
you find yourself.

—Unknown

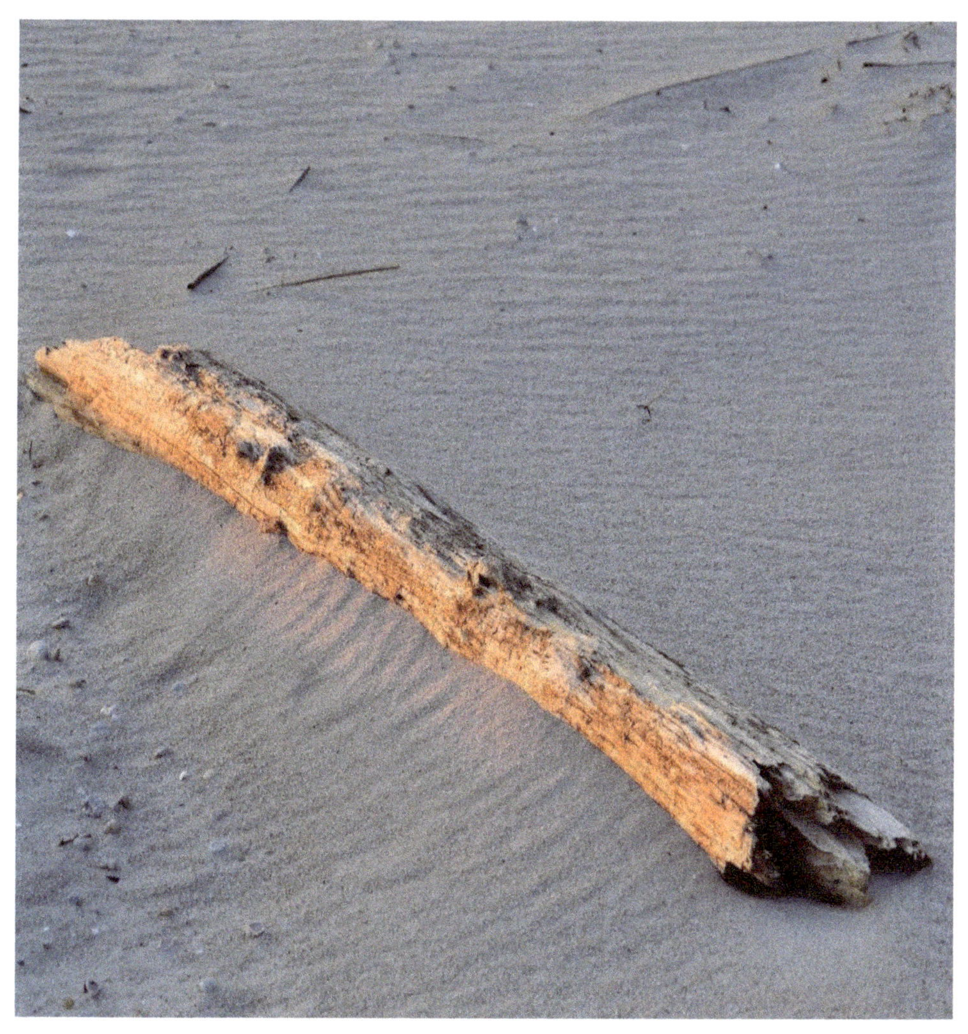

A life that hasn't a definite plan
is likely to become driftwood.

—David Sarnoff

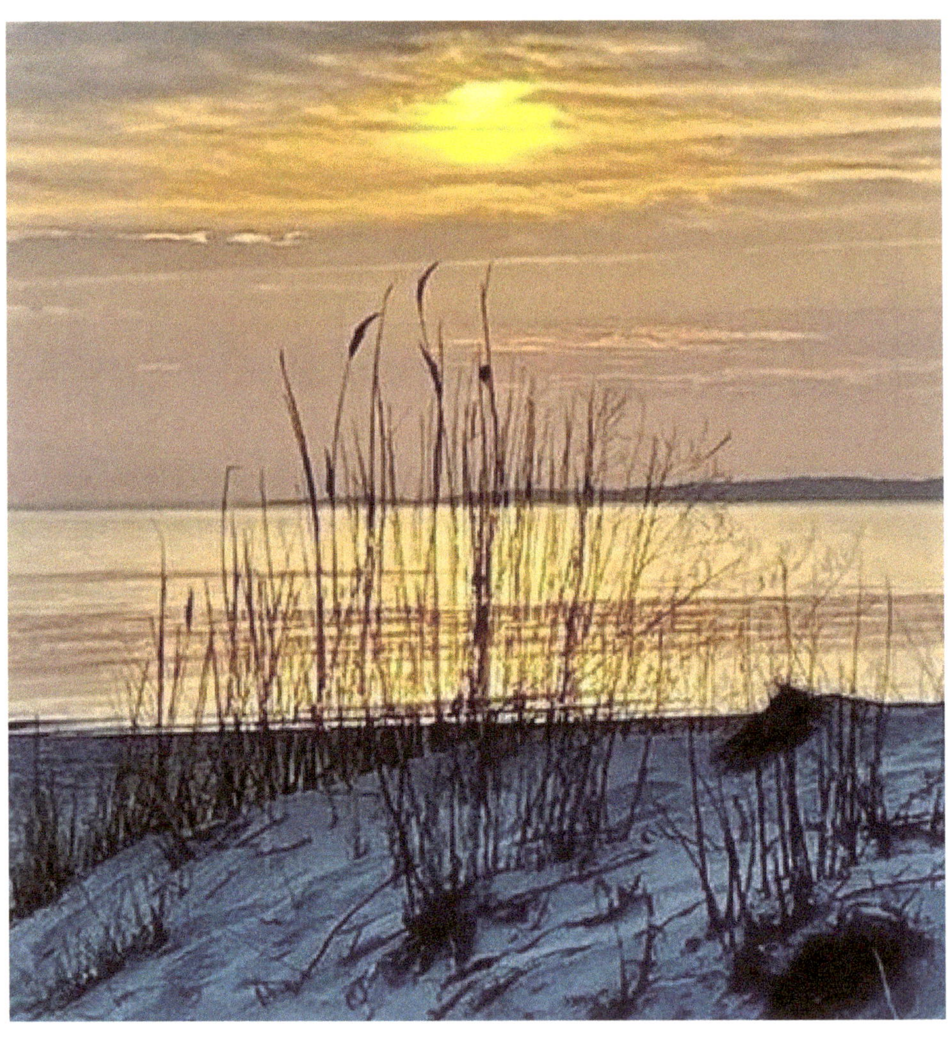

The key to success is not what you do,
it is how you feel about what you are doing.

—Iyanla Vanzant

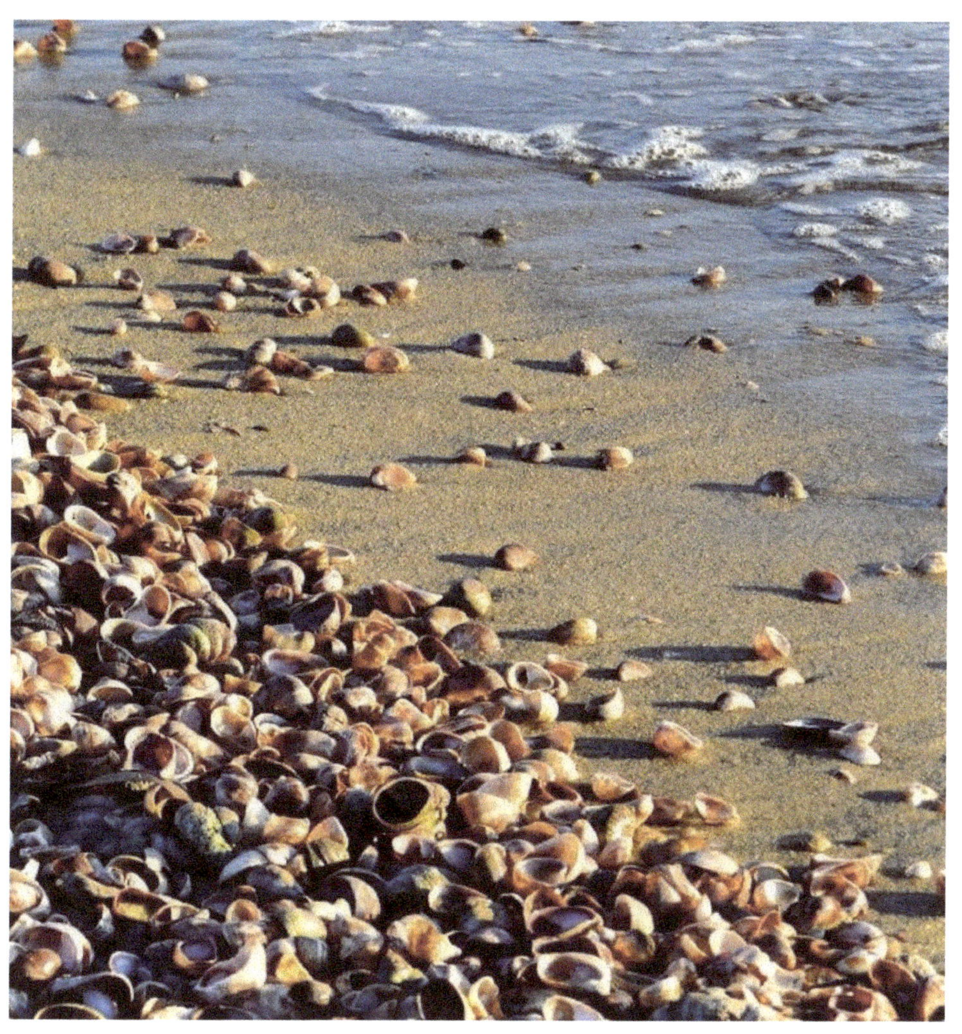

The shell, a reminder we're not meant
to be in one place.

—Deb Johnson

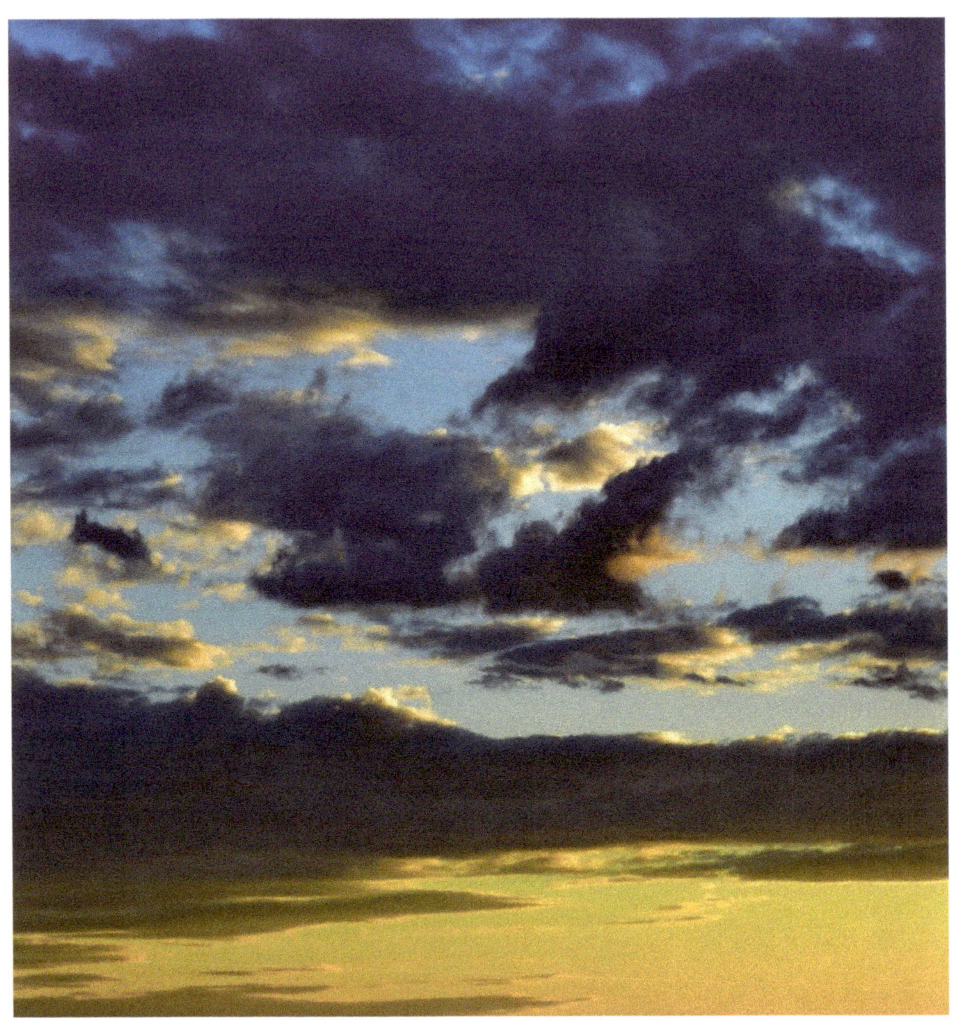

Dreams are the window to your future.
The goals are the vehicle that get you there.

—Sugar Ray Leonard

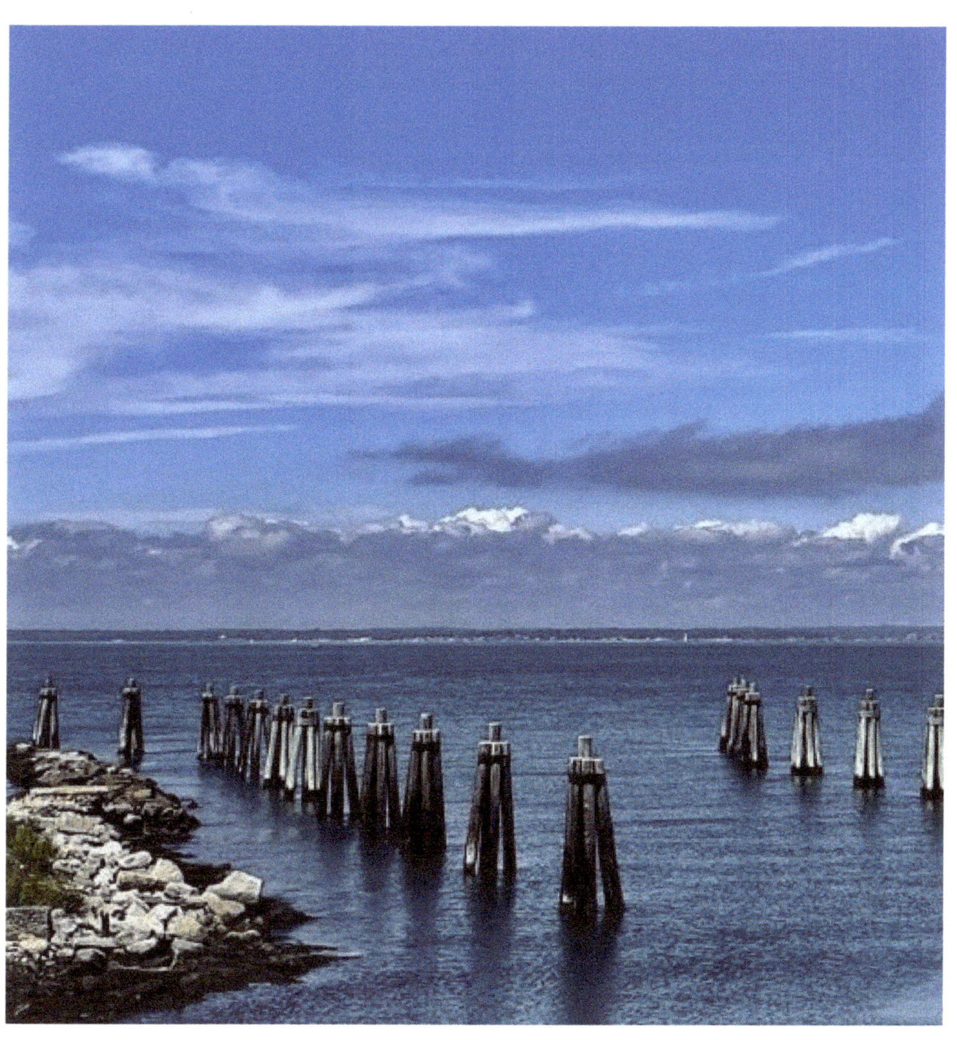

Life is like a river—it keeps flowing,
flowing and flowing till it merges into the Sea.
Nothing can stop the flow of Life,
but you can enjoy the Journey...

—RVM

CHAPTER 7

Keeping a Strong Work Ethic

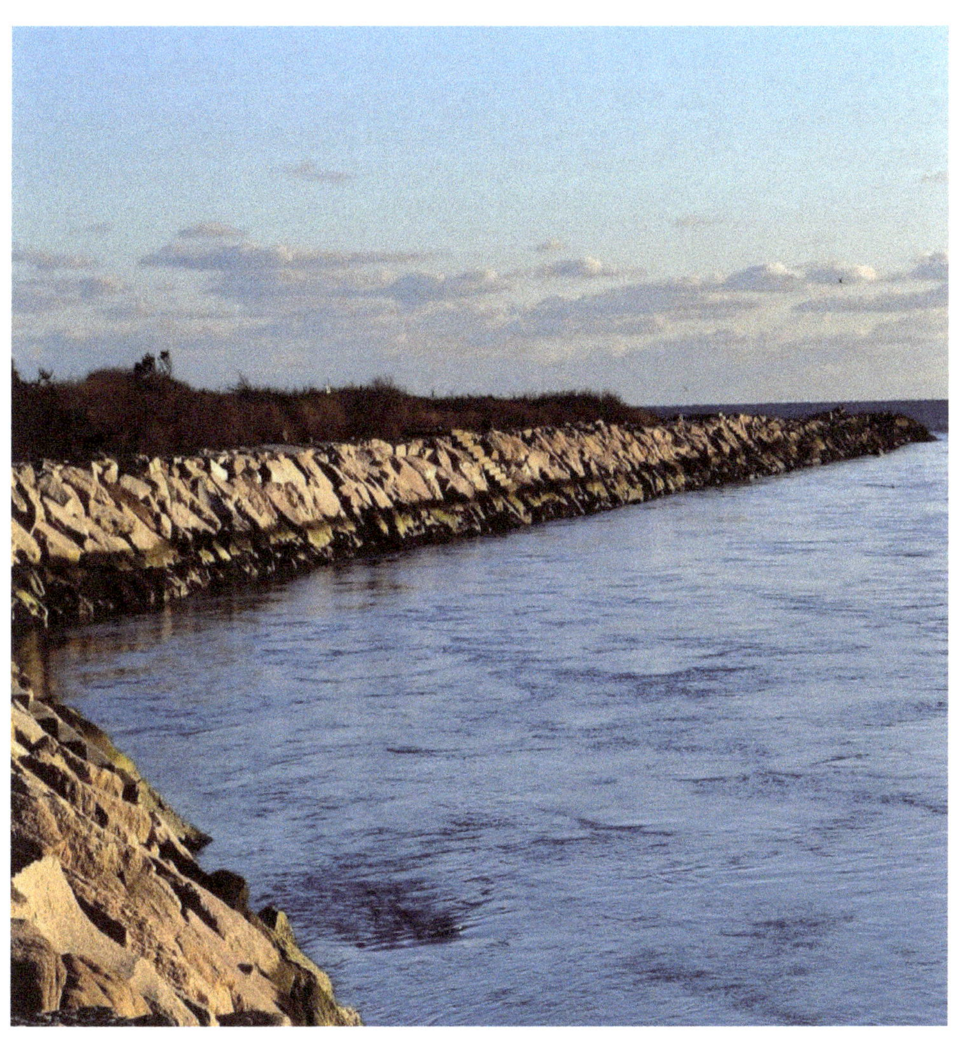

Don't wait for things to get easier, simpler, better.
Life will always be complicated.
Learn to be happy right now.
Otherwise, you'll run out of time.

—Unknown

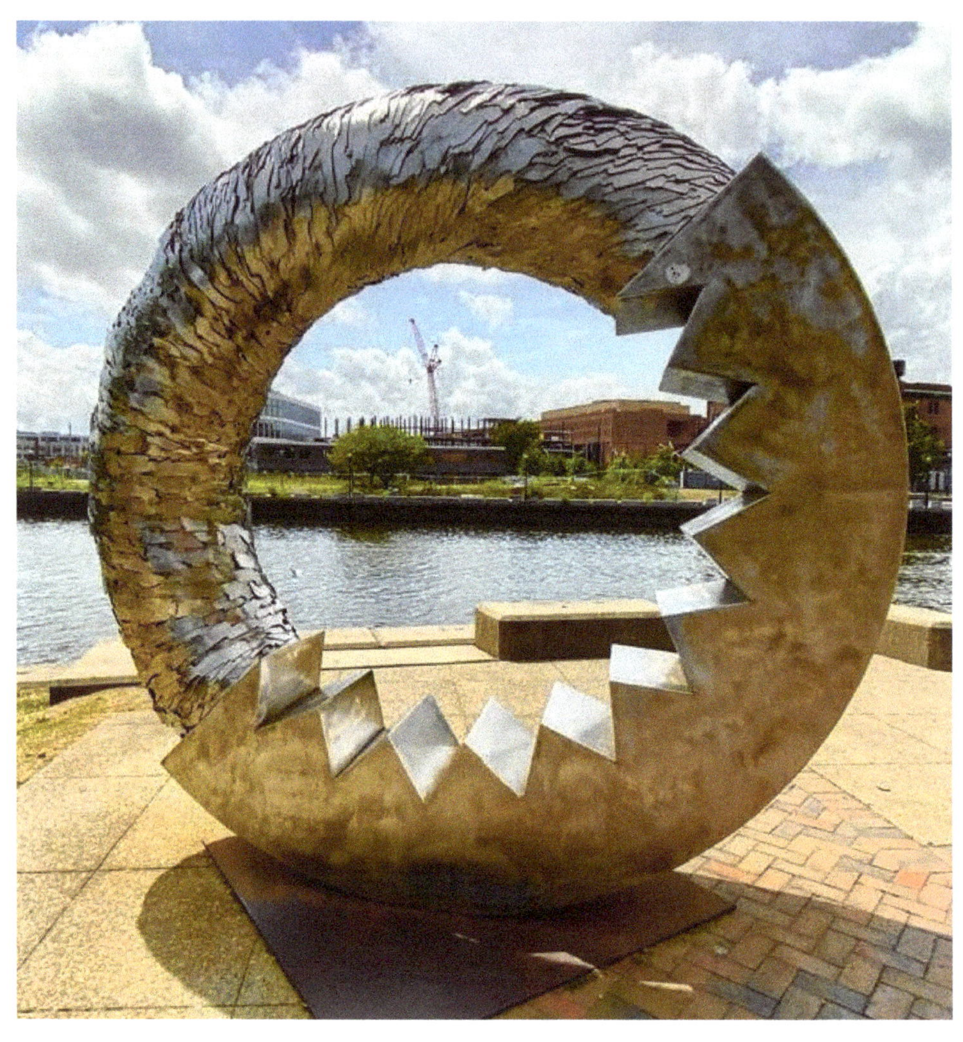

In life you don't get what you wish for,
you get what you work for.

—Dr. Daniel Milstein

Concentrate all your thoughts
upon the work at hand.
The sun's rays do not burn
until brought to a focus.

—Alexander Graham Bell

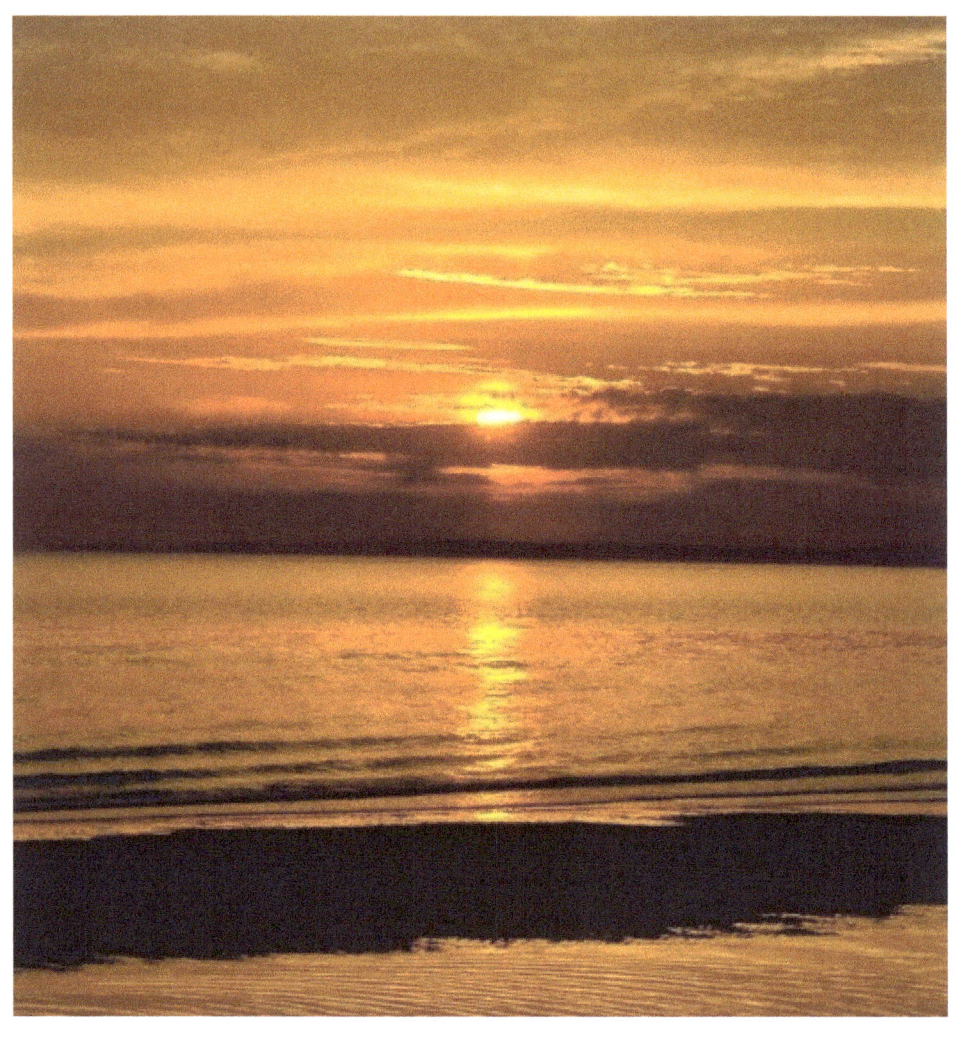

Doing the best at this moment puts you
in the best place for the next moment.

—Oprah Winfrey

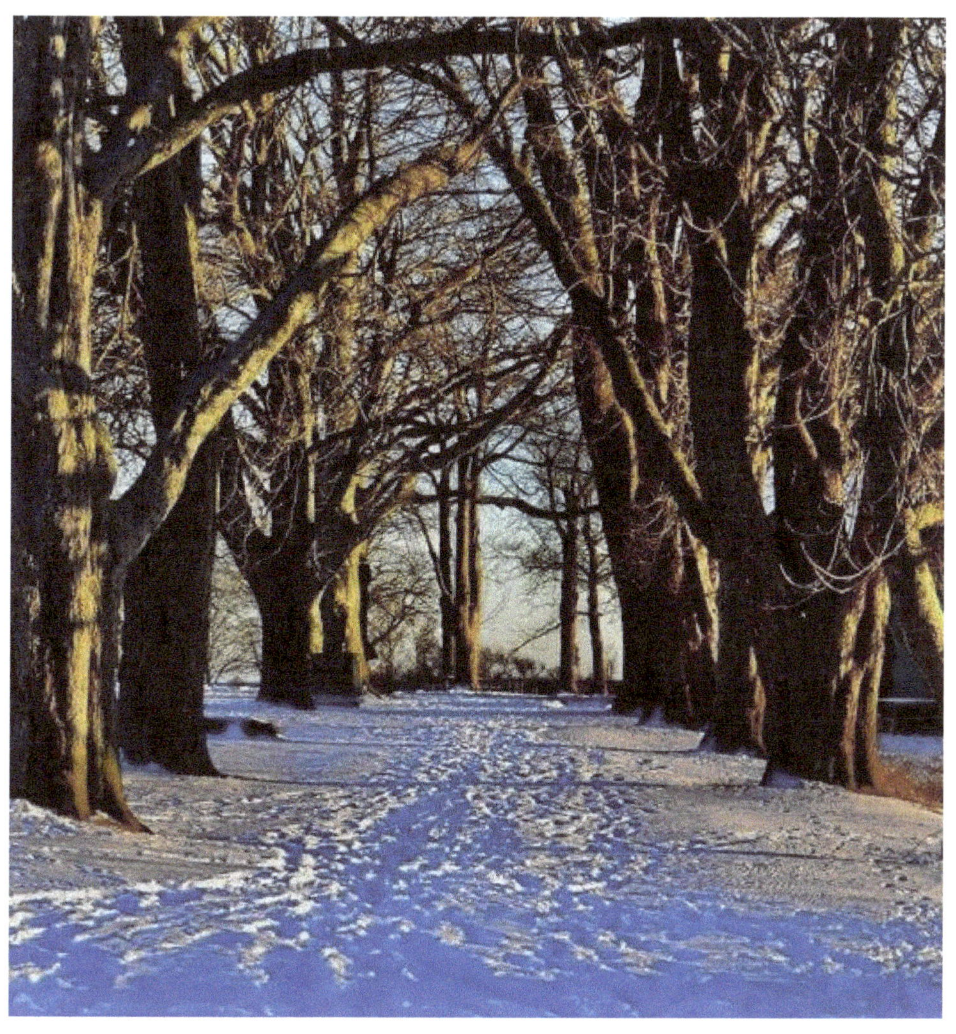

If you're walking down the right path
and you're willing to keep walking,
eventually you'll make progress.

—Barack Obama

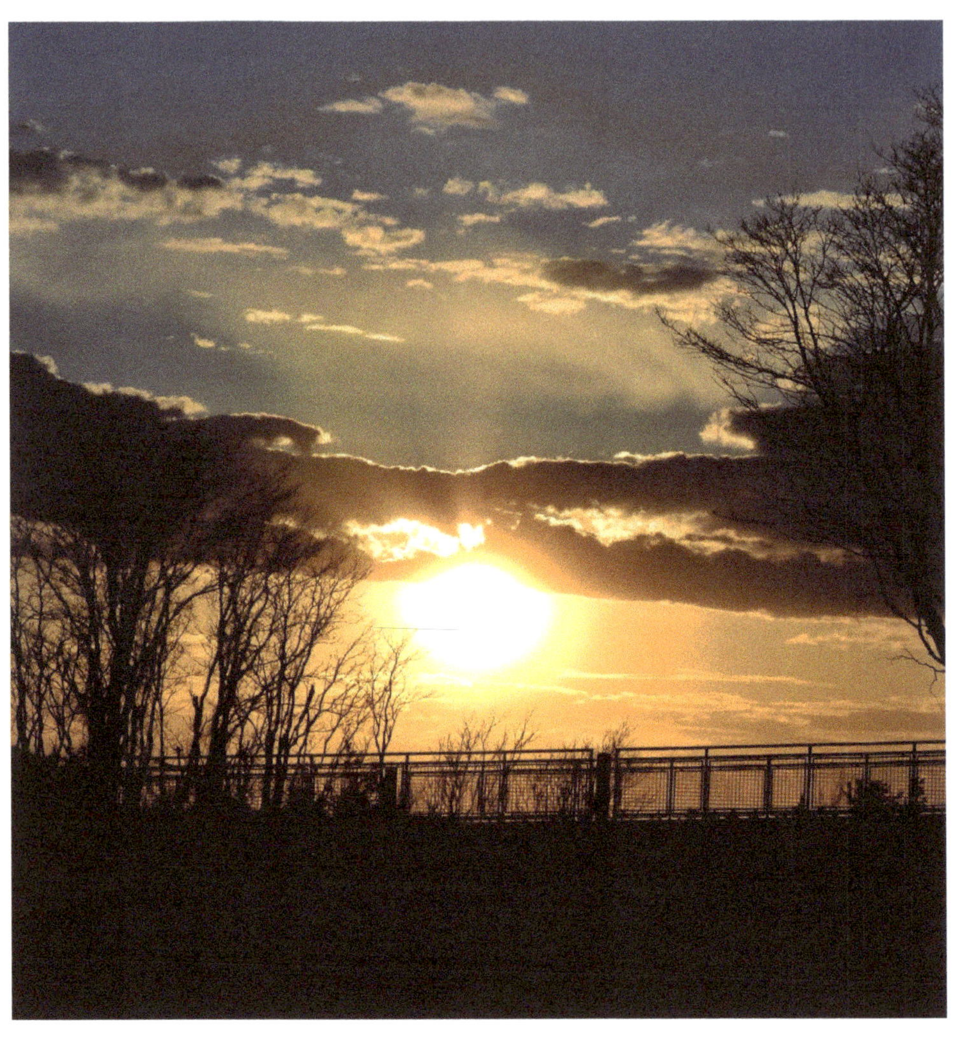

Distractions and excuses will always be there.
Opportunities won't.

—The Mindset Journey

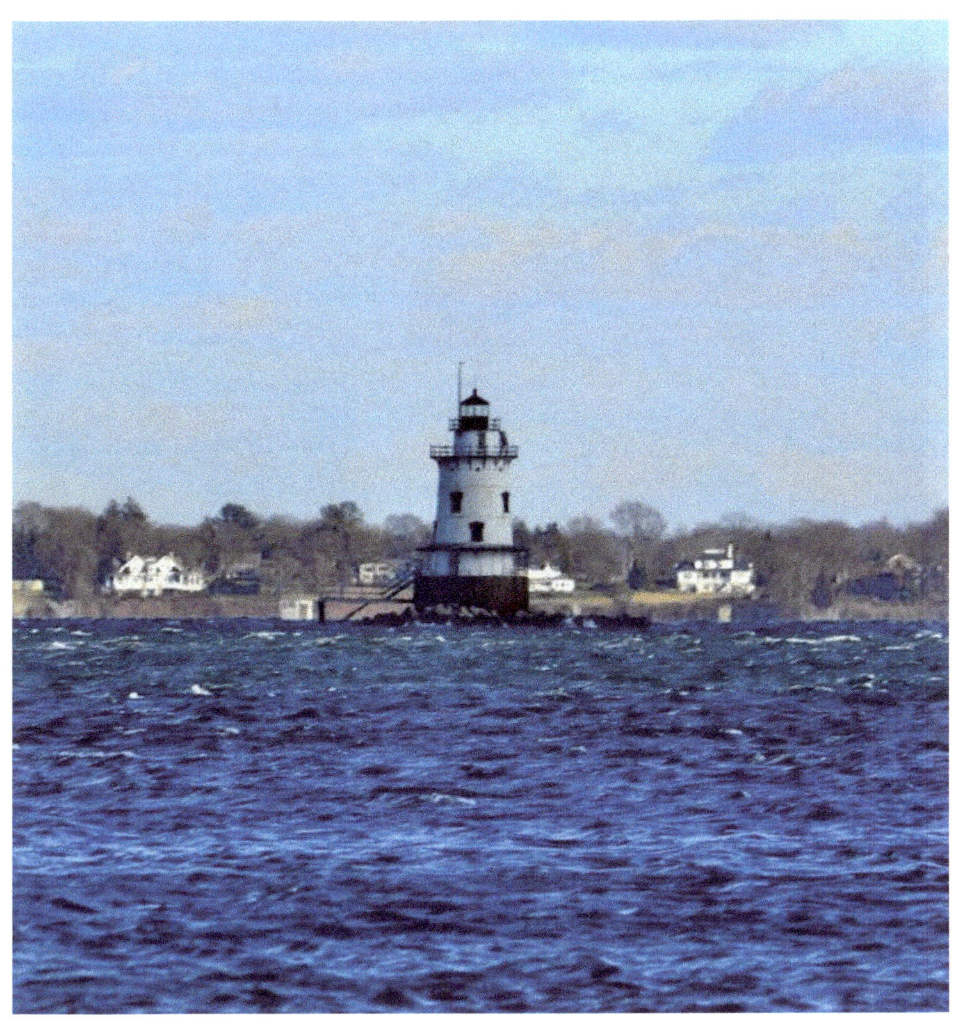

Man must behave like a lighthouse;
he must shine day and night
for the goodness of everyman.

—Mehmet Murat ildan

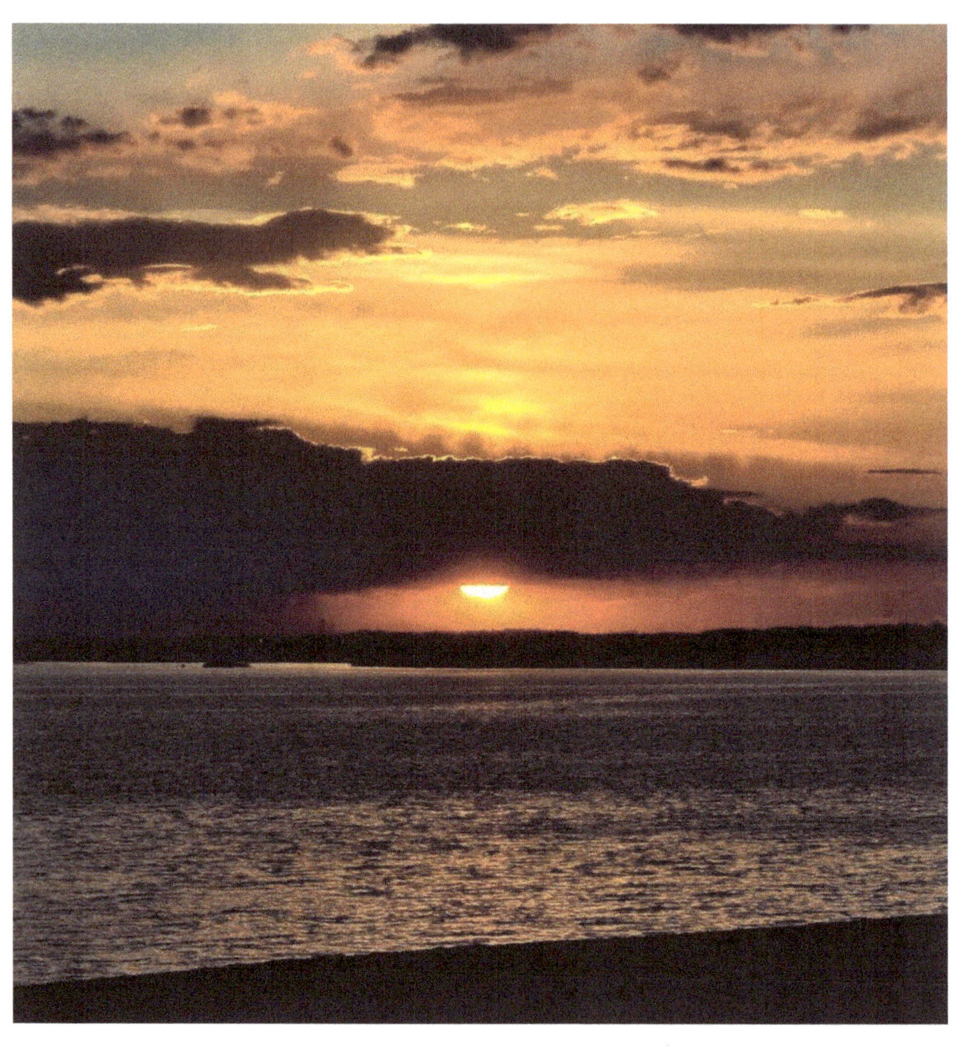

Commitment means staying loyal to
what you said you were going to do
long after the mood you said it in has left you.

—Orebela Gbenga

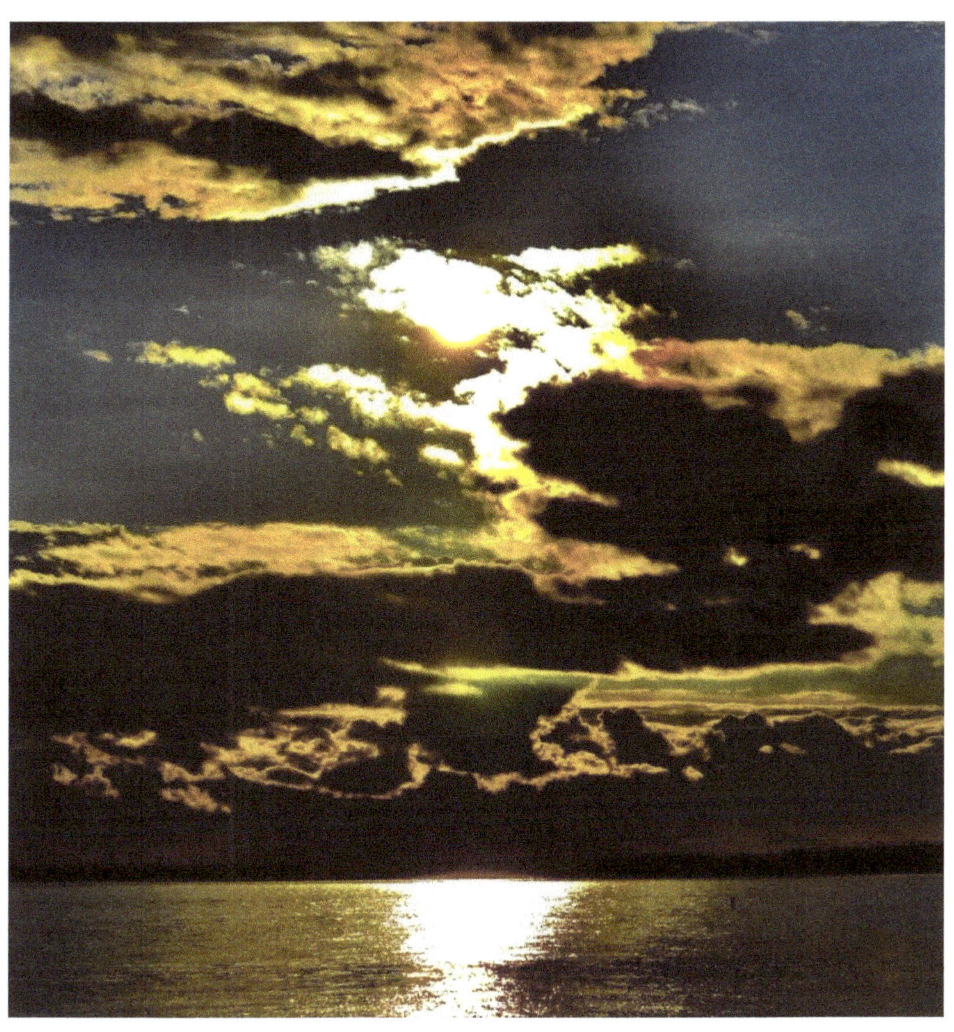

Success is the best revenge,
but revenge is not the best success.

—Davin Michael Stedman

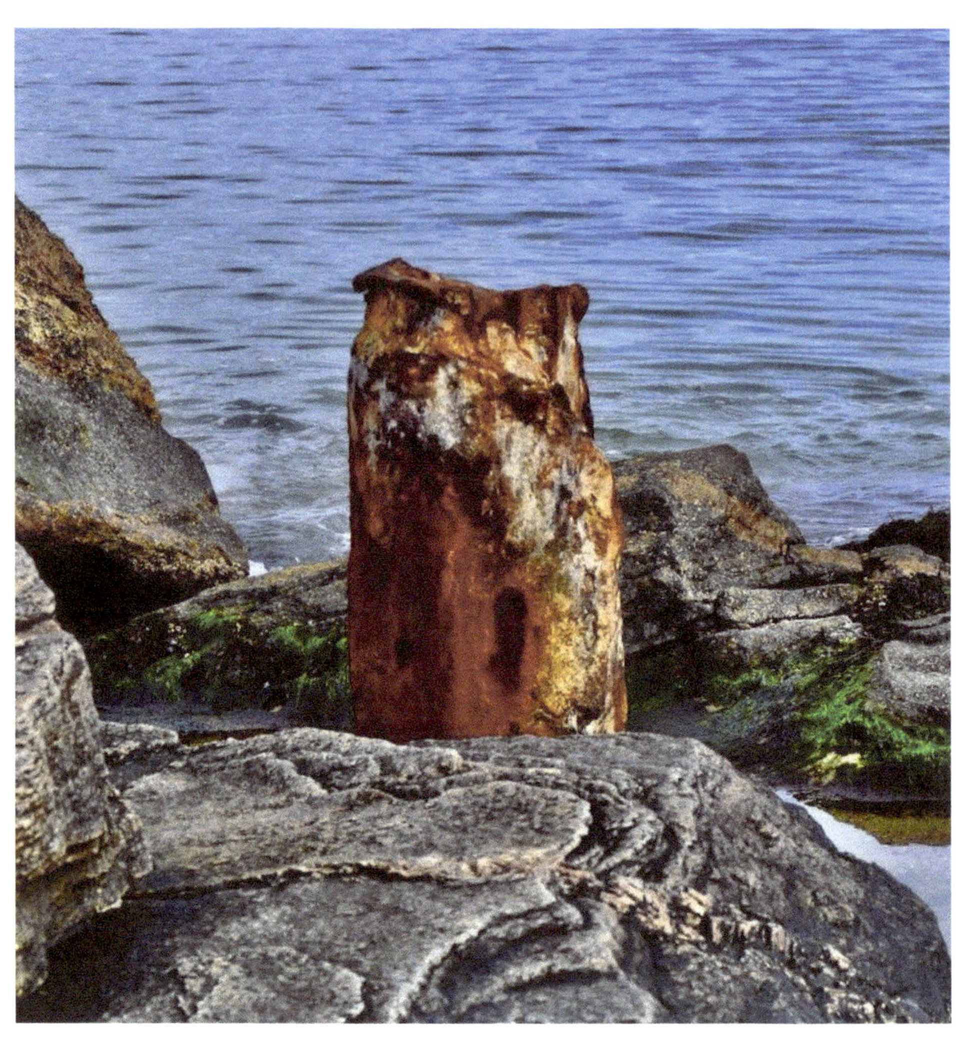

I'd much rather wear out than rust out.

—Dan Rather

CHAPTER 8

Overcoming Obstacles

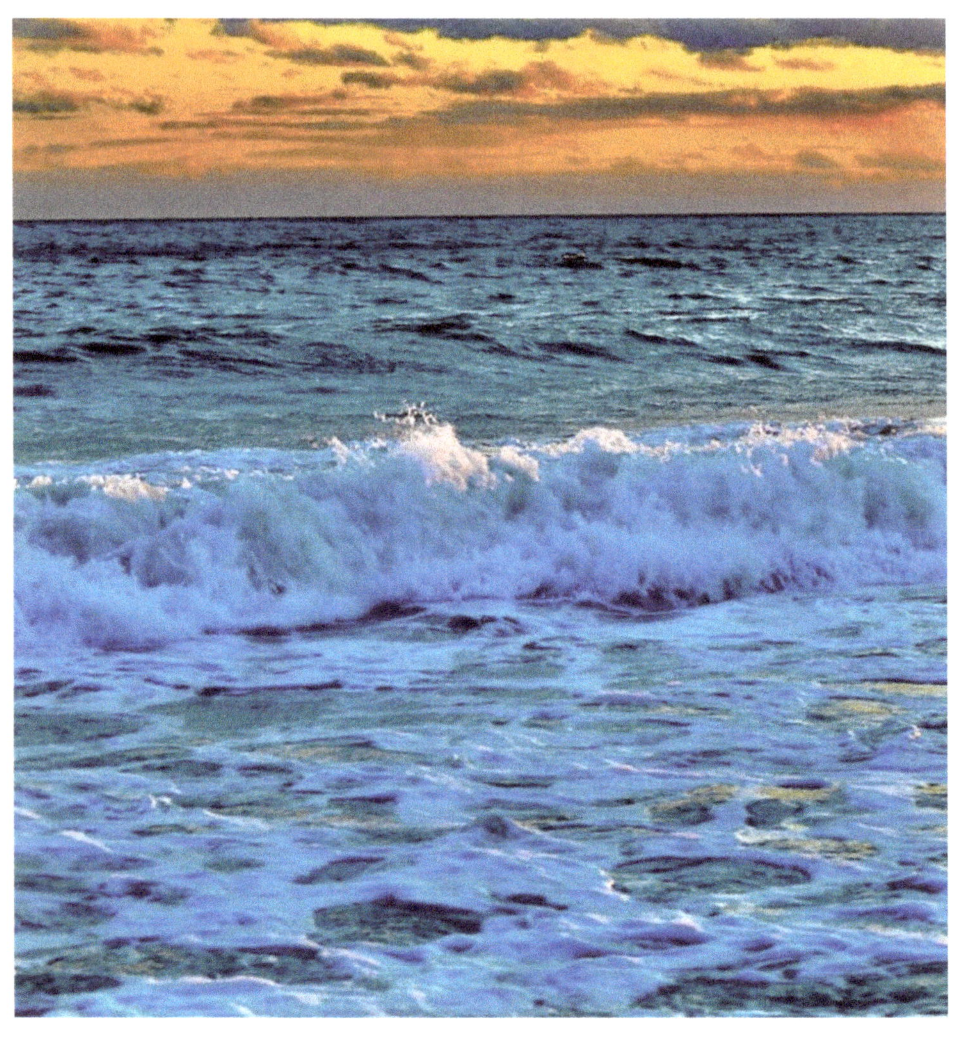

When something bad happens
you have three choices.
You can either let it define you, let it destroy you,
or you can let it strengthen you.

—Dr. Seuss

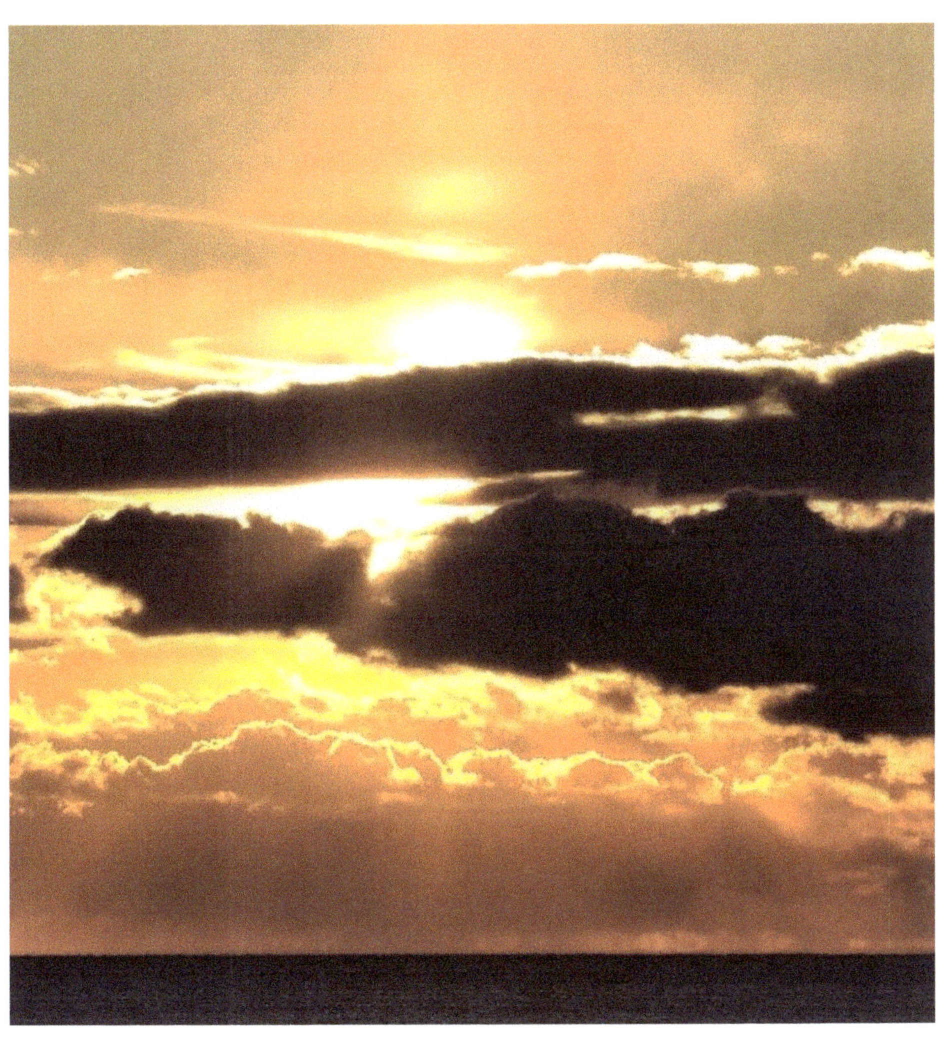

Not all storms come to disrupt your life,
some come to clear your path.

—Paolo Coelho

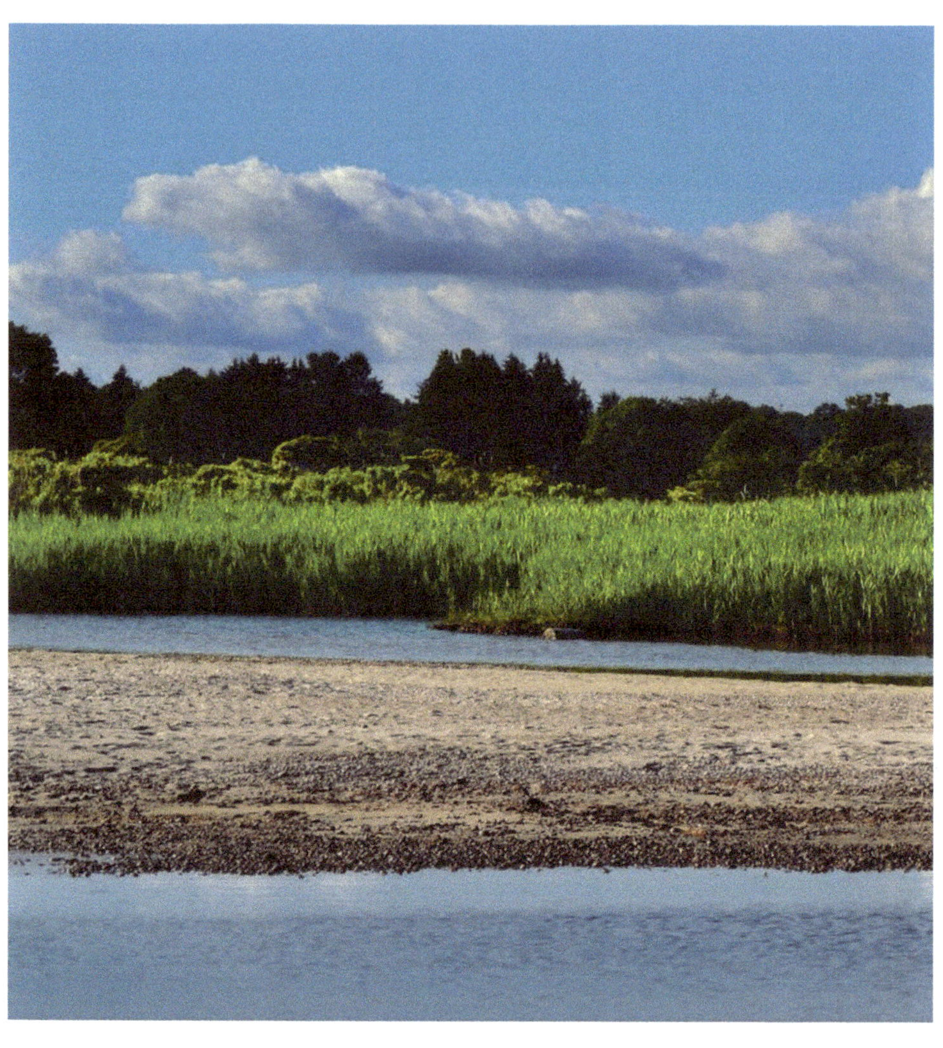

Not every person is going to understand you and that's ok. They have a right to their opinion and you have every right to ignore it.

—Joel Osteen

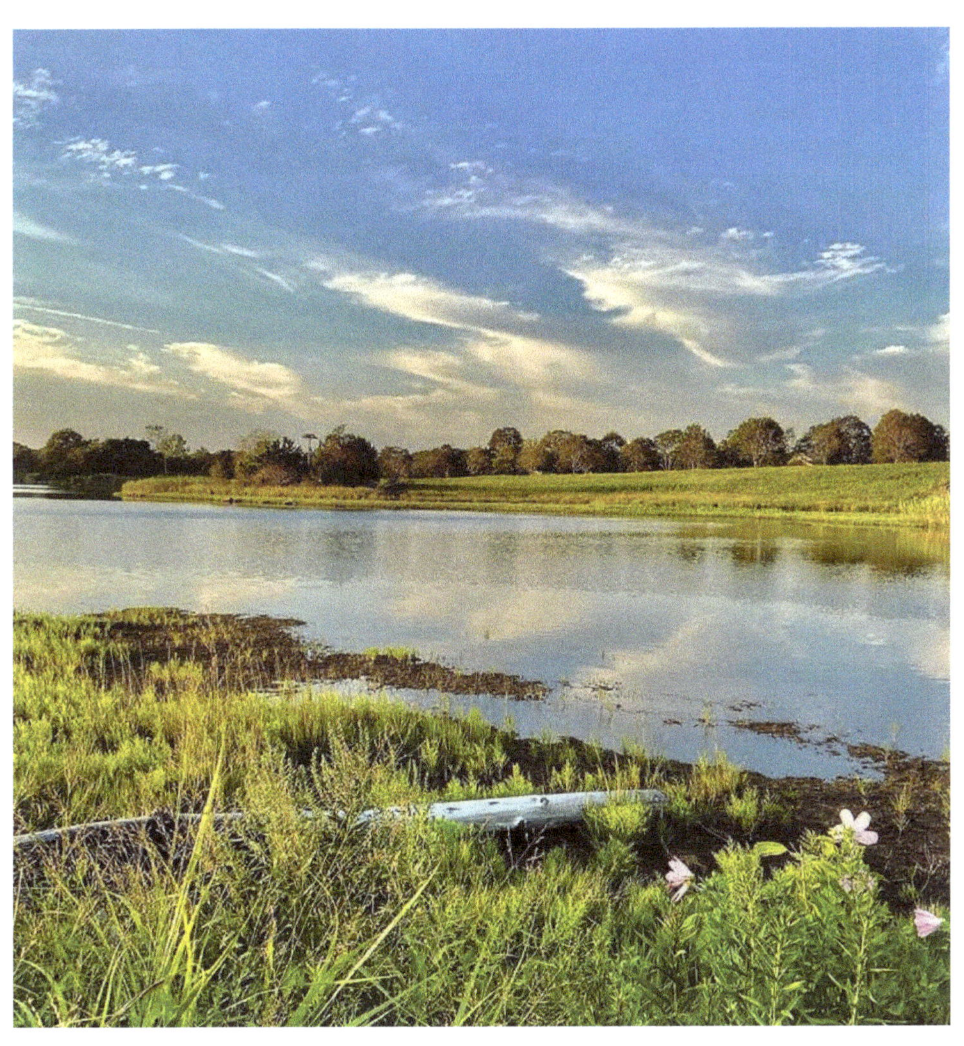

You don't always have to tell your side of the story. Time will.

—Anuj Setia

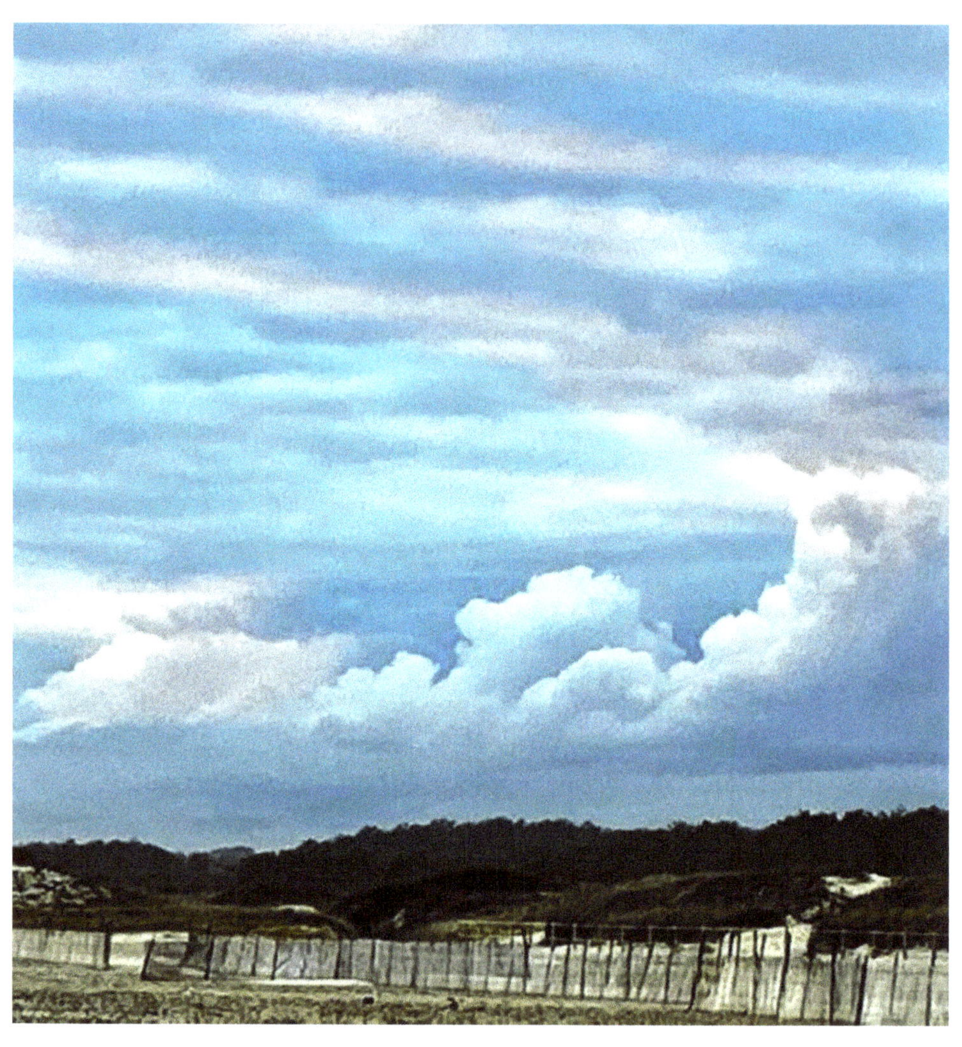

When we feel stuck, look at the sky.
The clouds remind us that everything changes.

—Unknown

Healing yourself is connected
with healing others.

—Yoko Ono

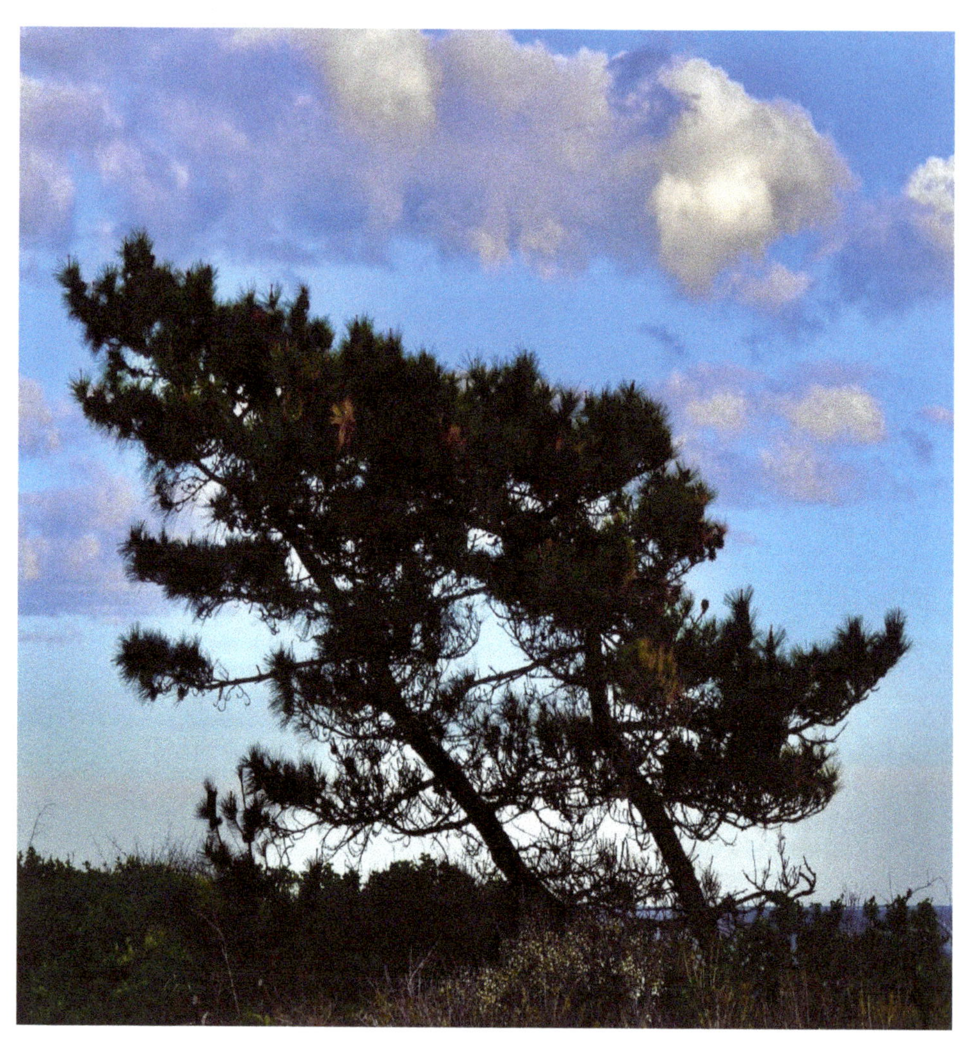

Live life as if everything is rigged in your favor.

—Rumi

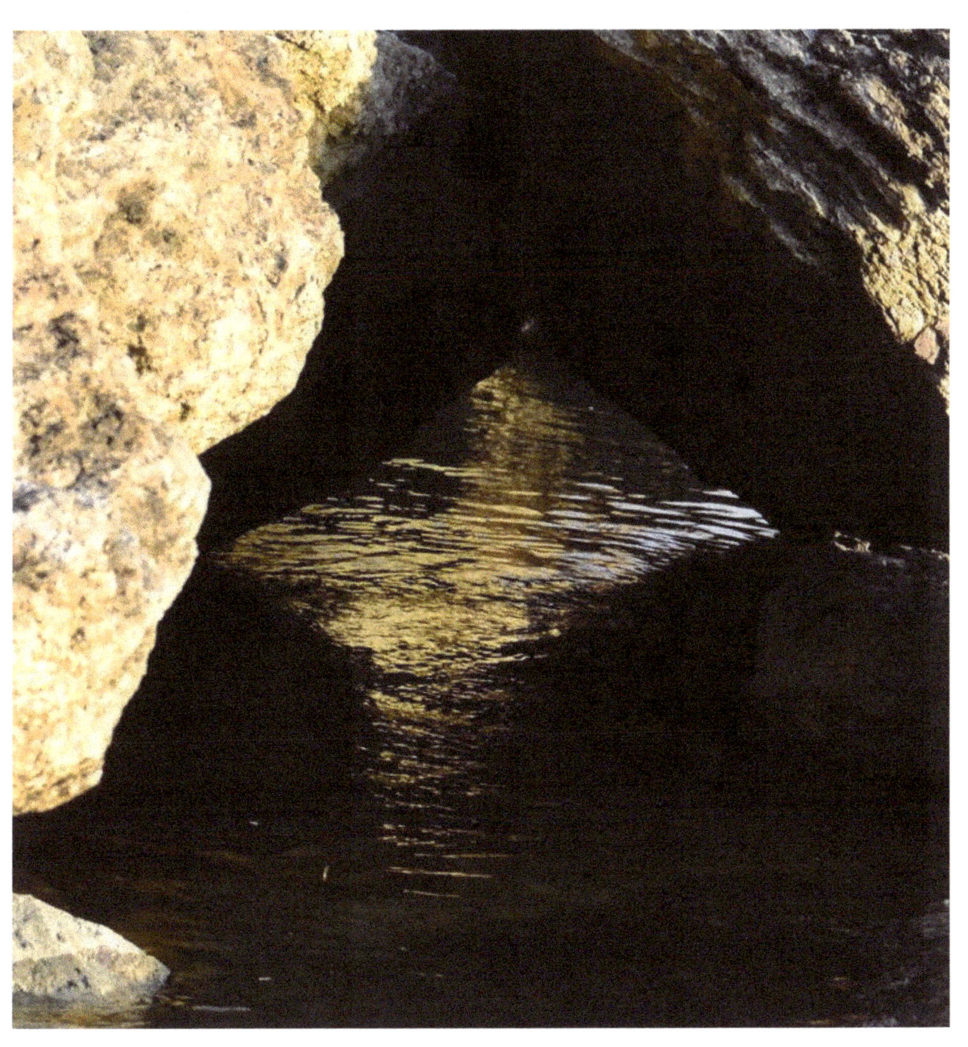

Flow like water.
Even the largest rocks may stand in its way,
water will always find a way to get through.

—Roger Lee

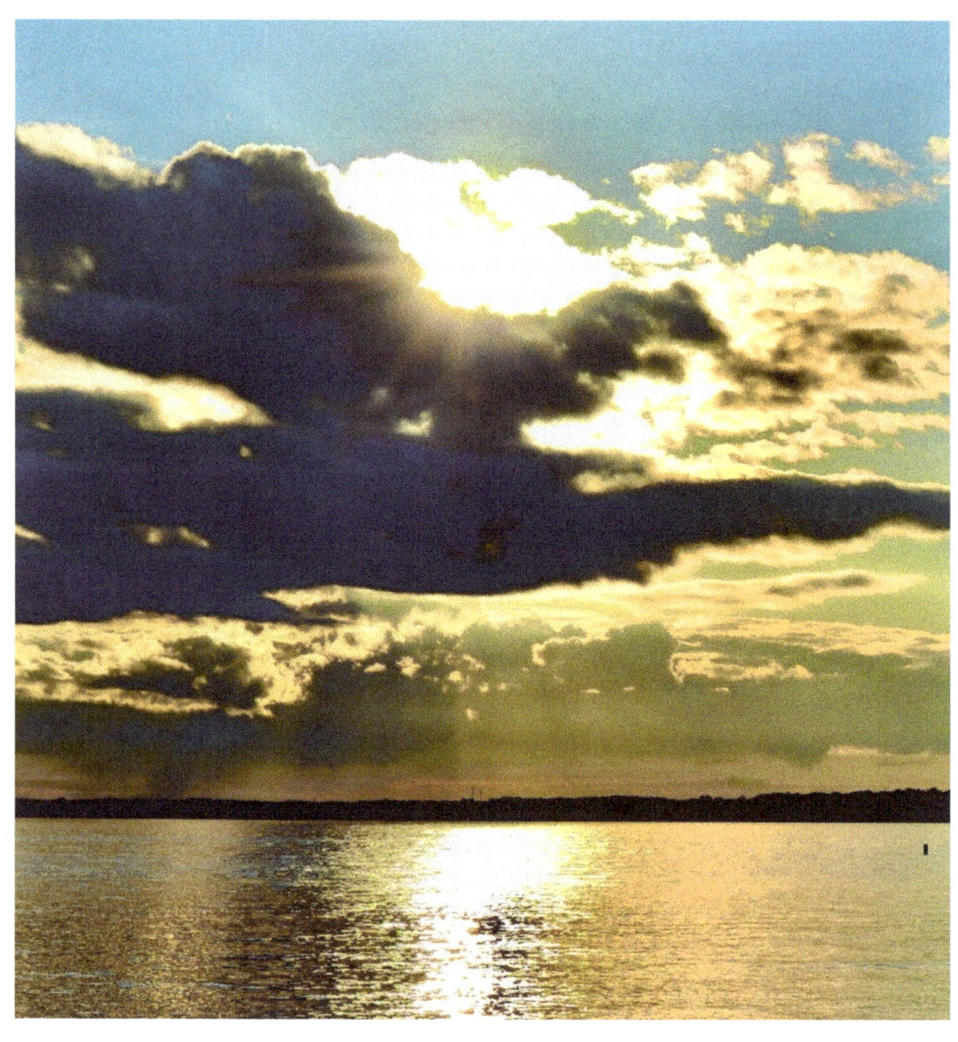

As the sun hides behind clouds,
success hides behind trouble.

—Matshona T. Dhilwayo

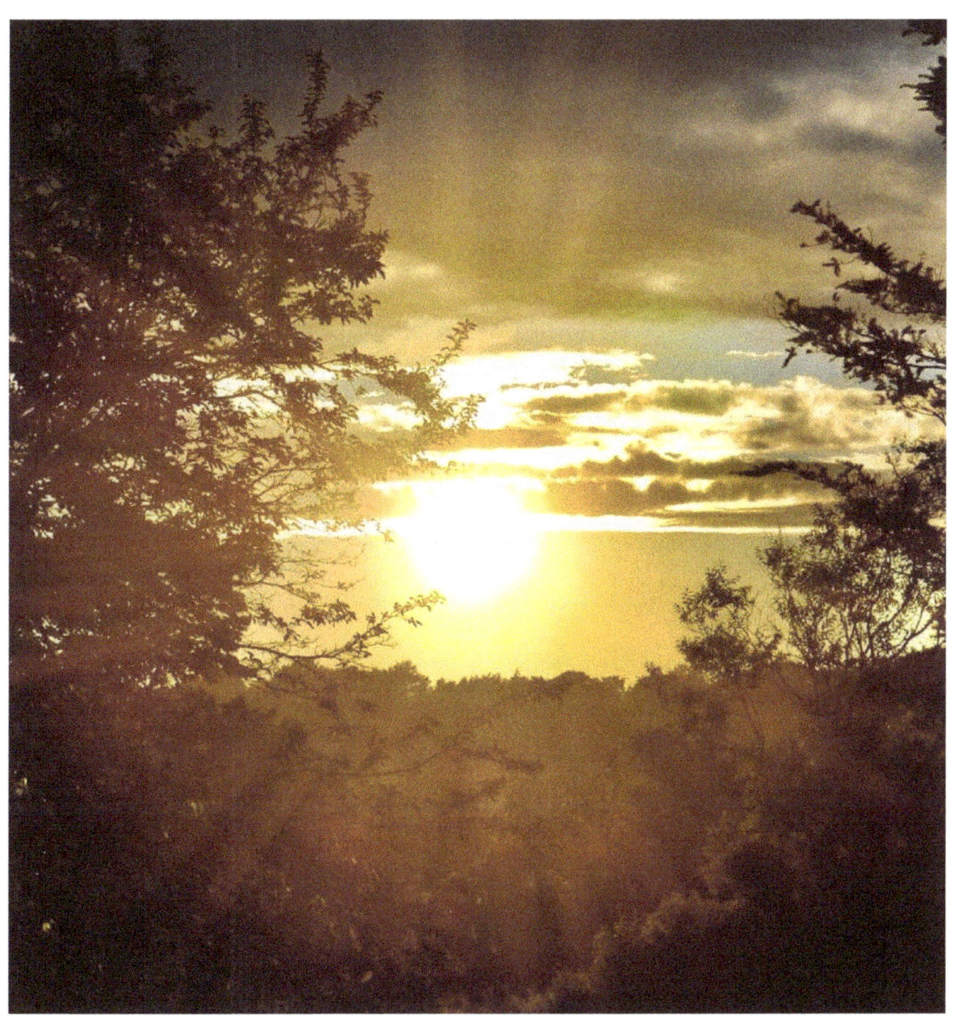

Life is not a problem to be solved,
but a reality to be experienced.

—Soren Kierkegaard

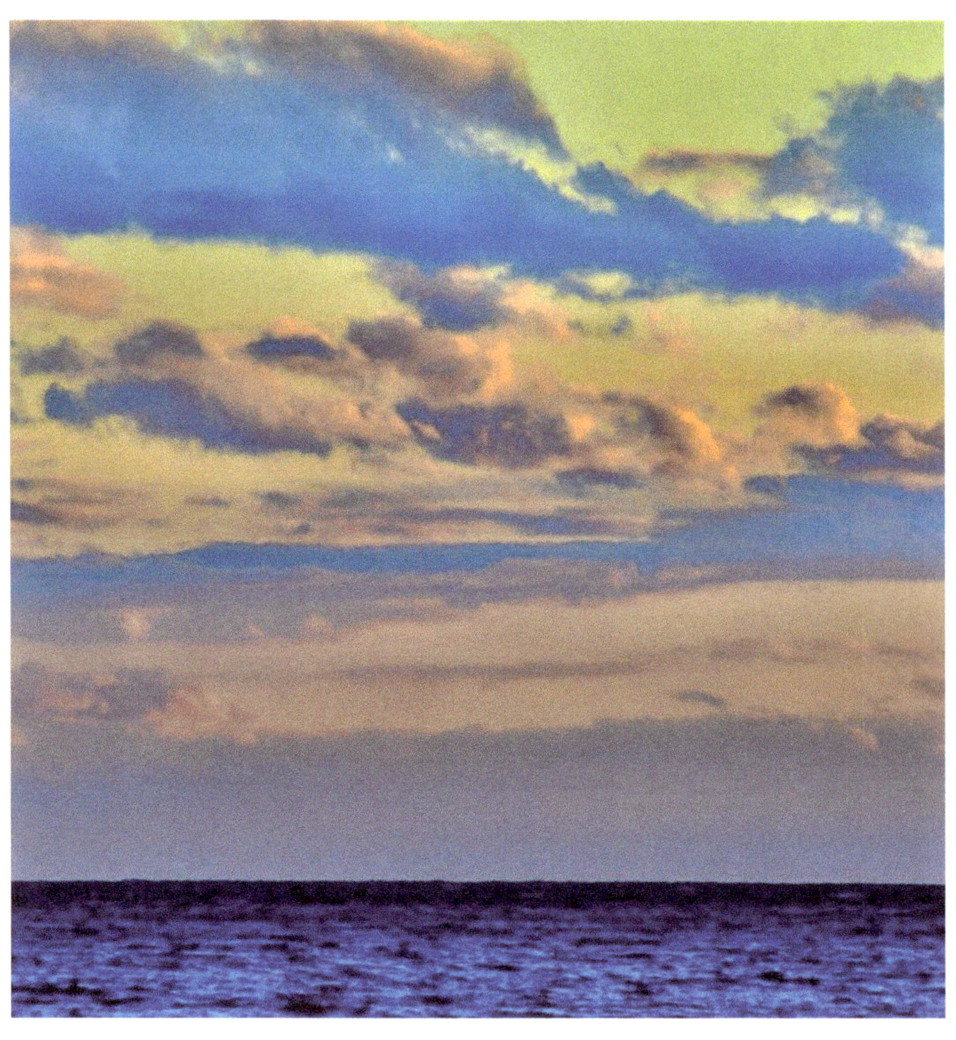

When something goes wrong in your life,
just yell "Plot twist!" and move on!

—Unknown

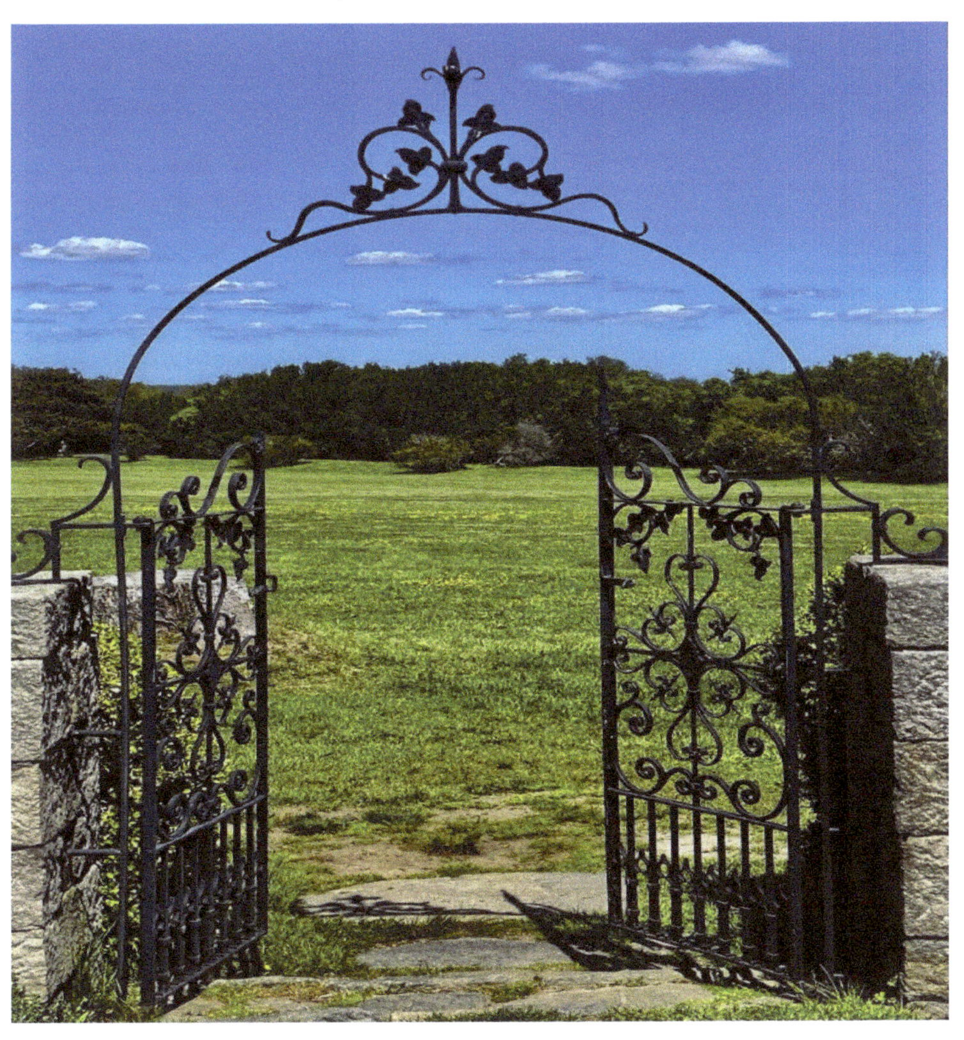

The longest part of the journey is said to be
the passing of the gate.

—Marcus Terentius Varro

CHAPTER 9

Making Tough Decisions

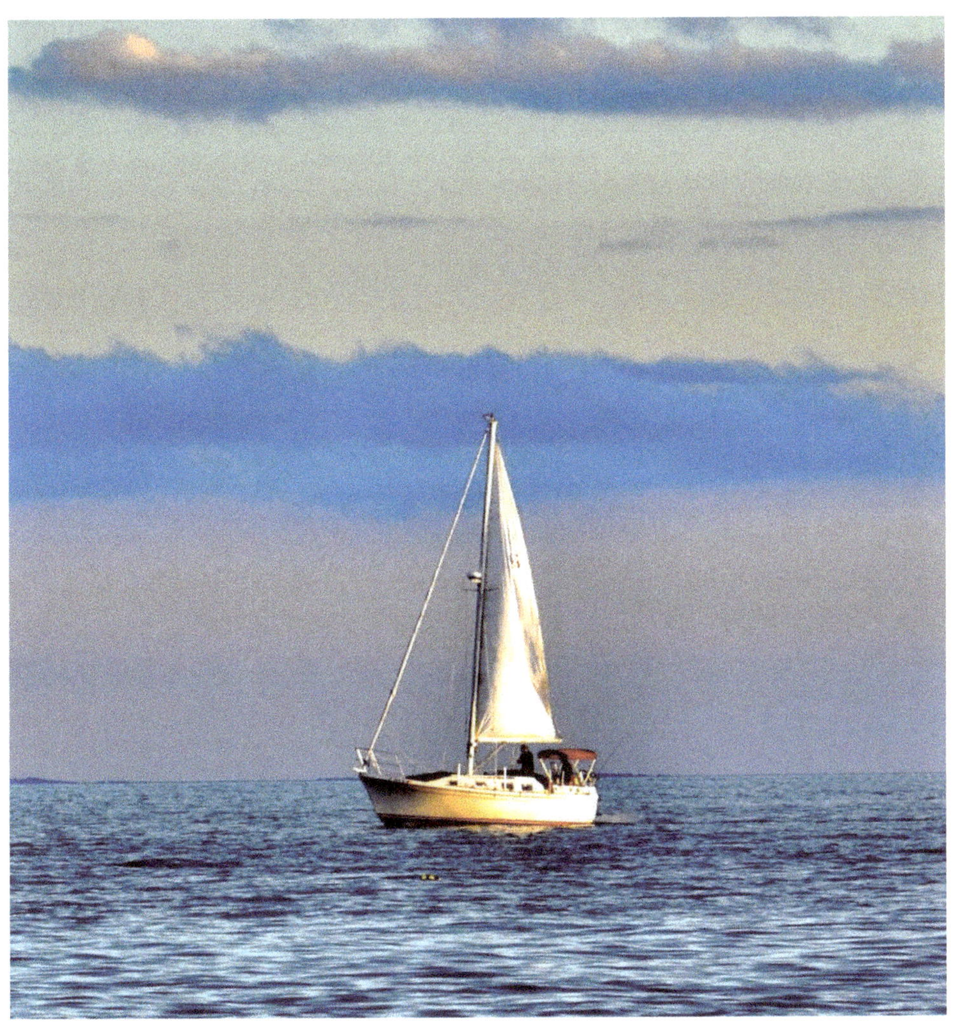

We can't control the winds,
but we can adjust our sails.

—Thomas S. Monson

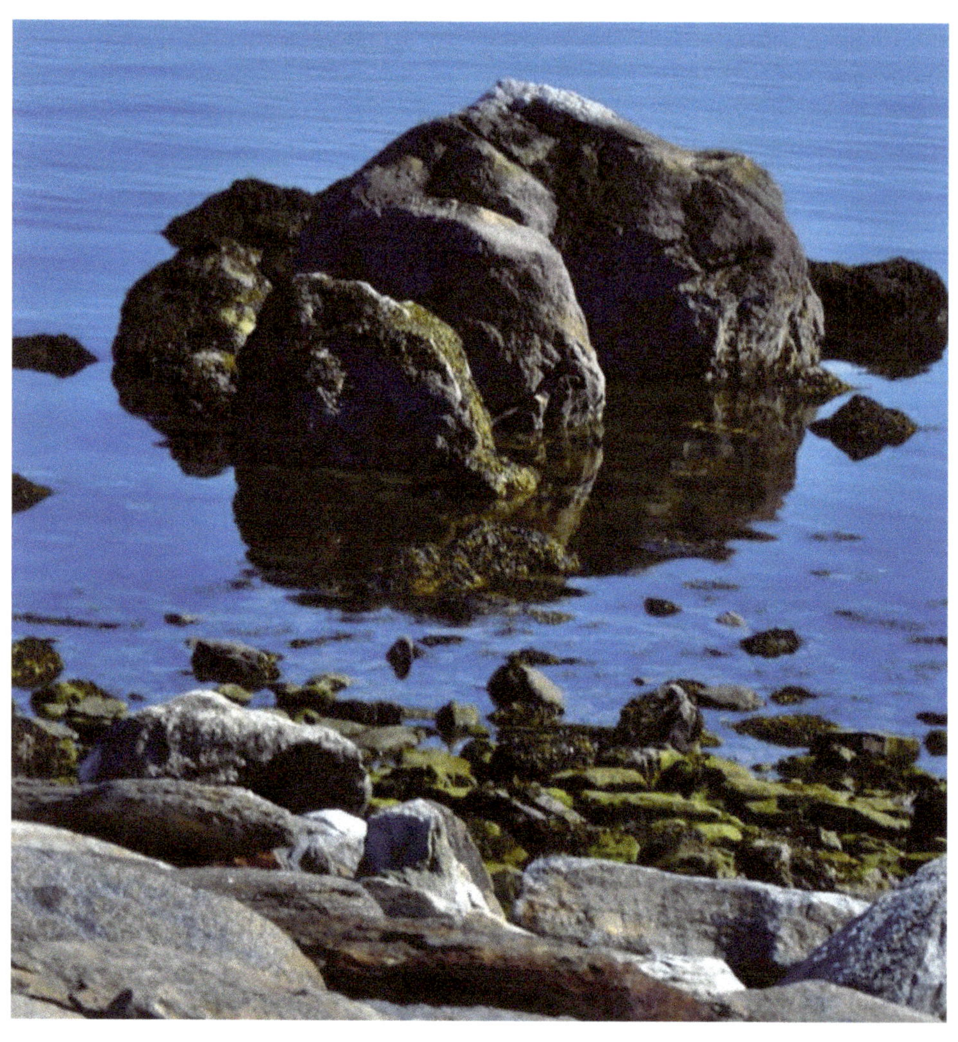

In matters of style, swim with the current;
in matters of principle, stand like a rock.

—Thomas Jefferson

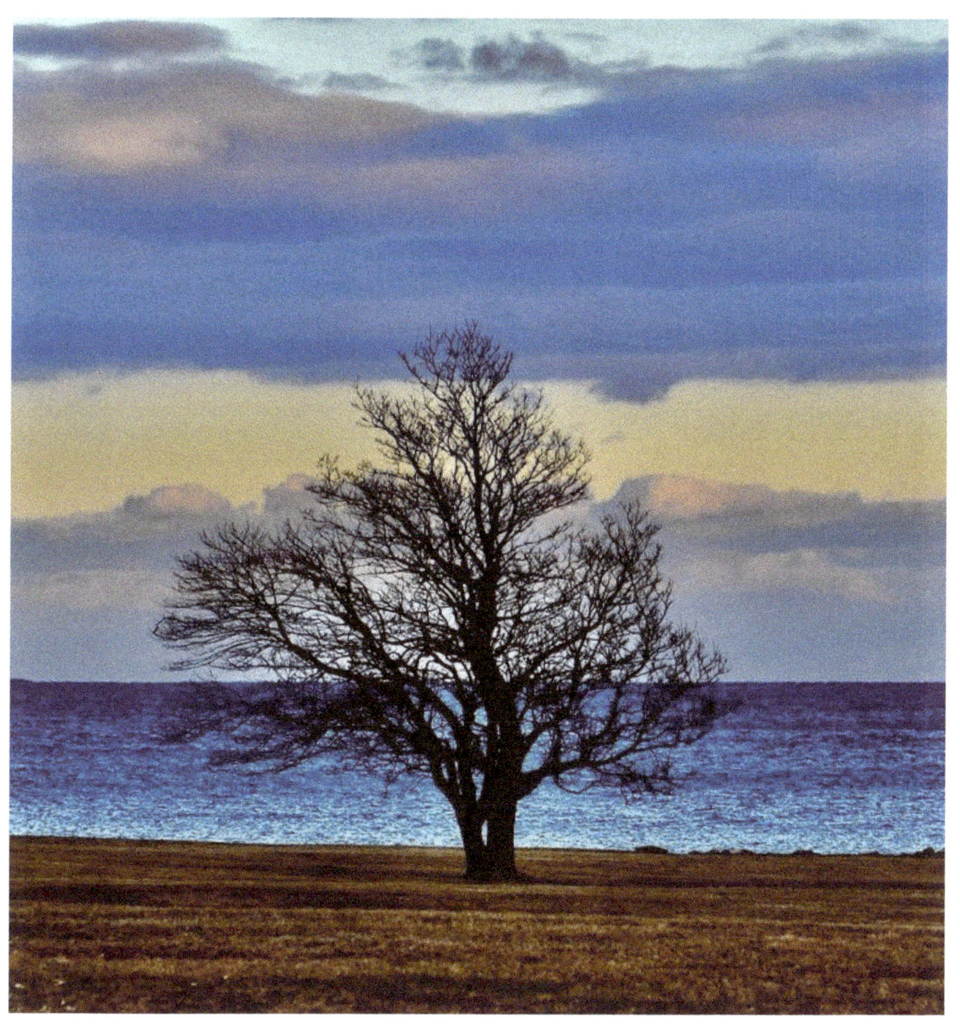

You have to stand for what you believe in
and sometimes you have to stand alone.

—Queen Latifah

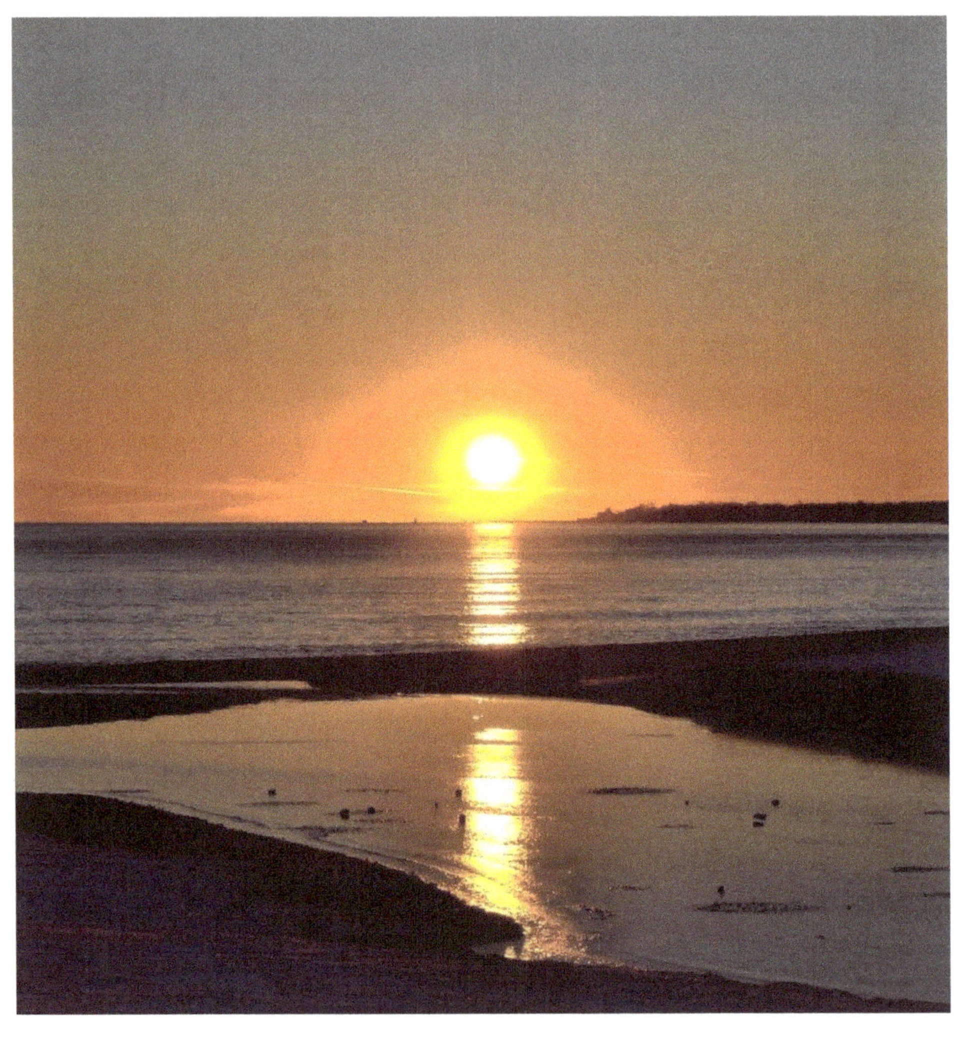

Everything in your life is a reflection of a choice you have made. If you want a different result, make a different choice.

—Unknown

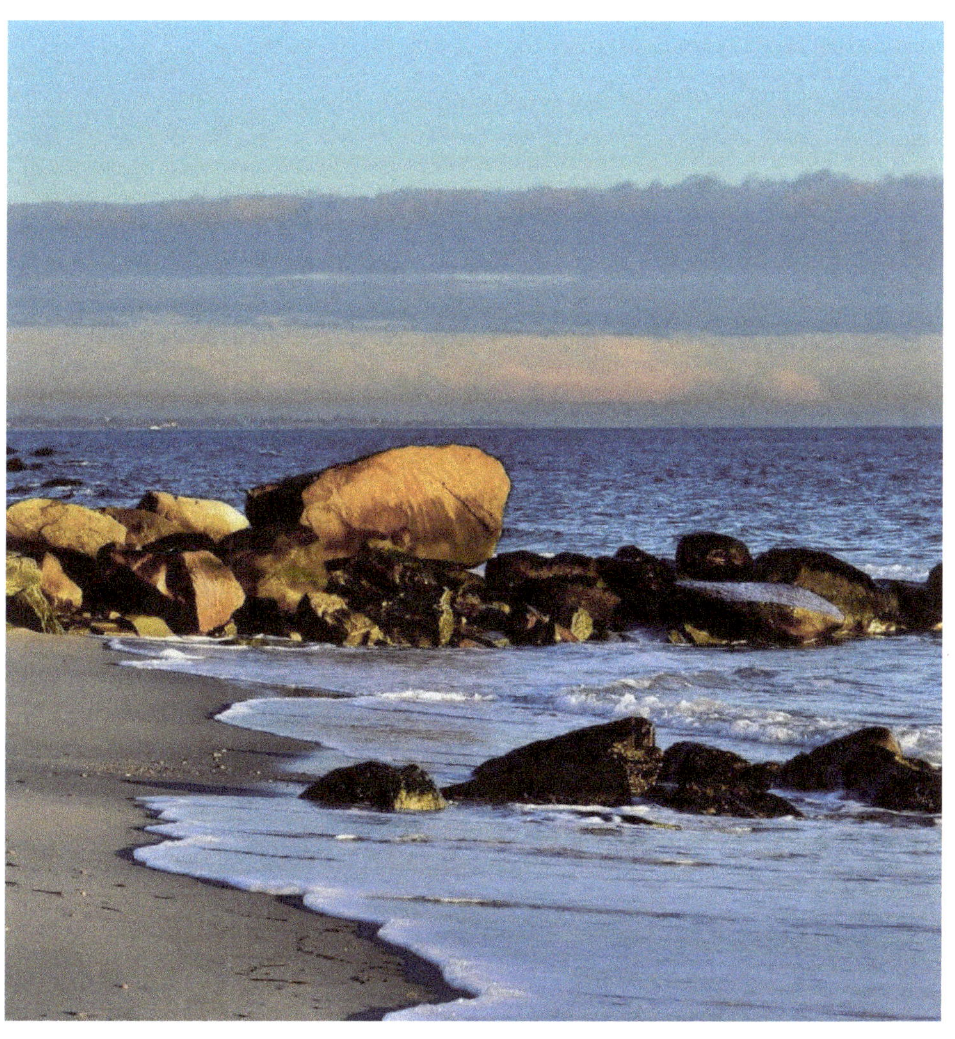

Make your decisions like a rock and
live your life like a flow of water.

—Arlin Sailesh Kapadia

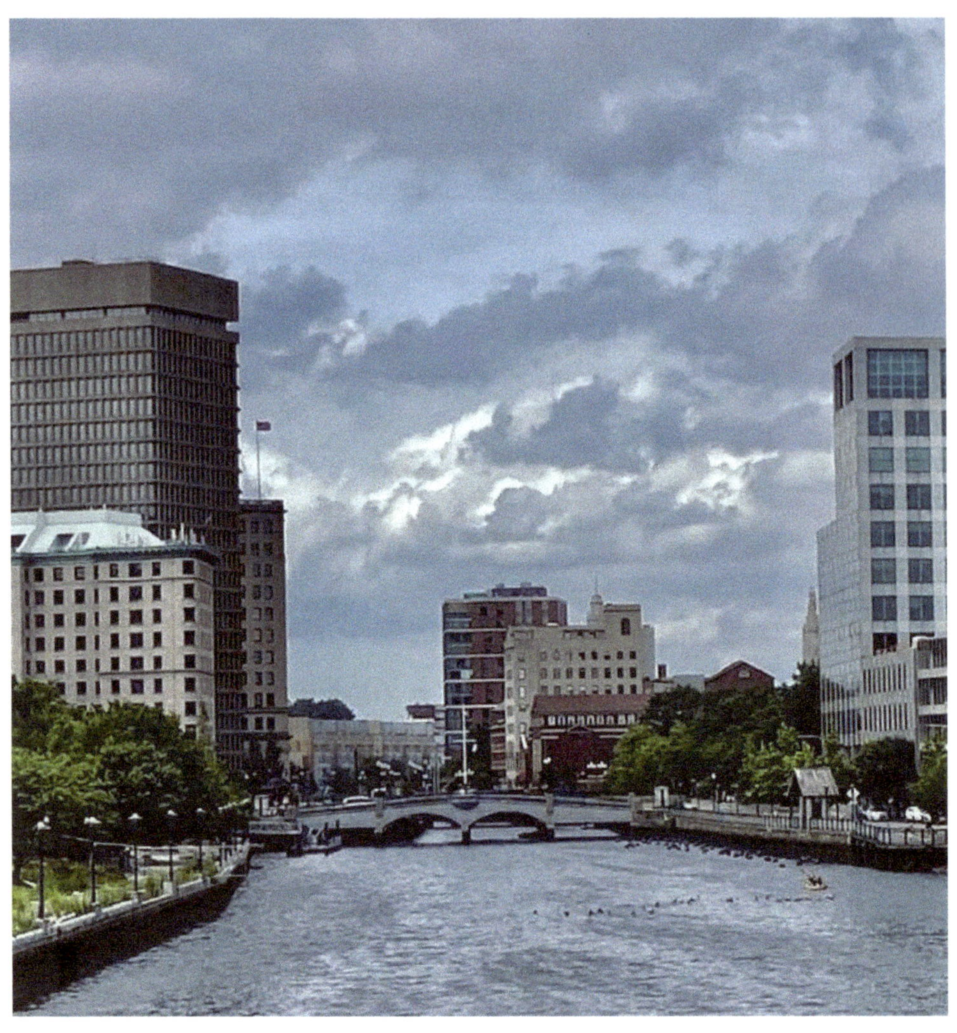

There comes a time when you have to stop crossing oceans for people who wouldn't even jump puddles for you.

—Unknown

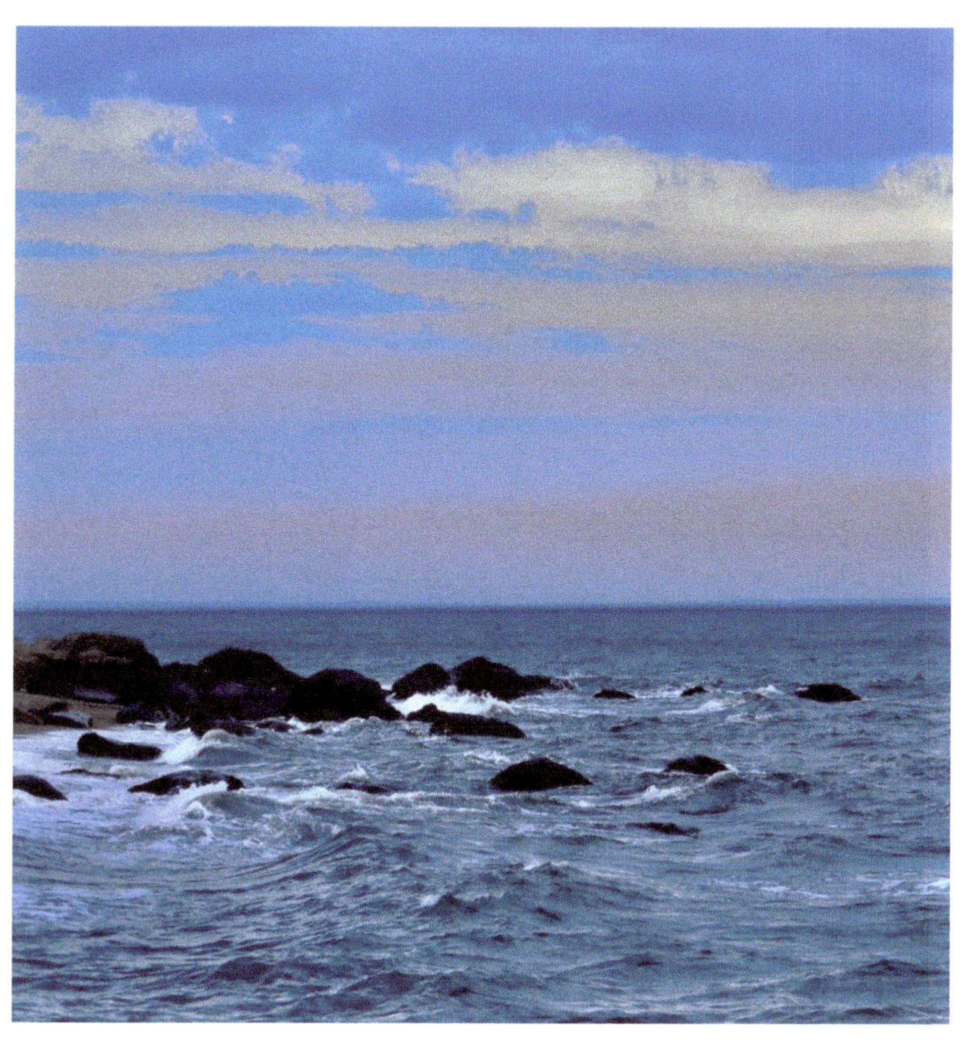

When you can't control what's happening,
challenge yourself to control the way
you respond to what's happening.
That's where your power is.

—Unknown

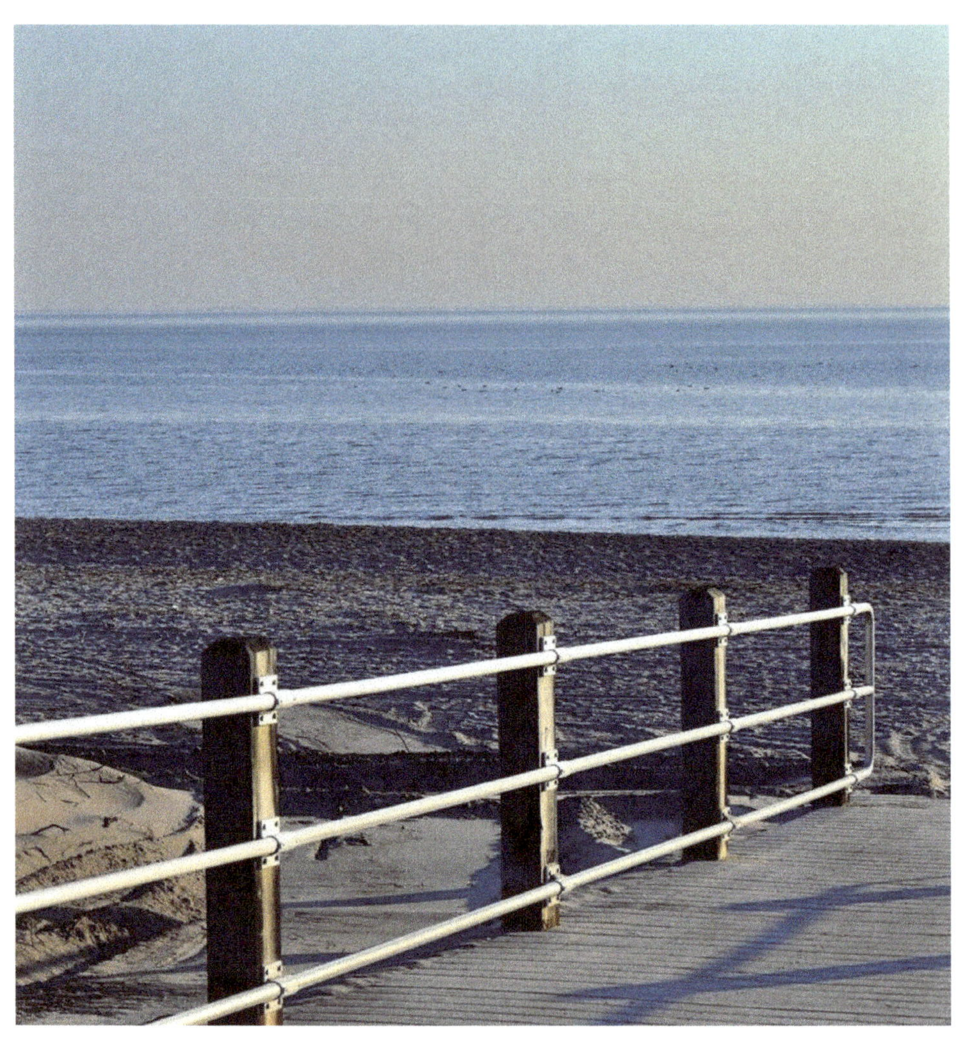

You can't keep a foot stuck in the past
if you're moving forward.
You'll never fully arrive at the
future that's waiting for you.

—Alfa

CHAPTER 10

Nurturing Social Connections

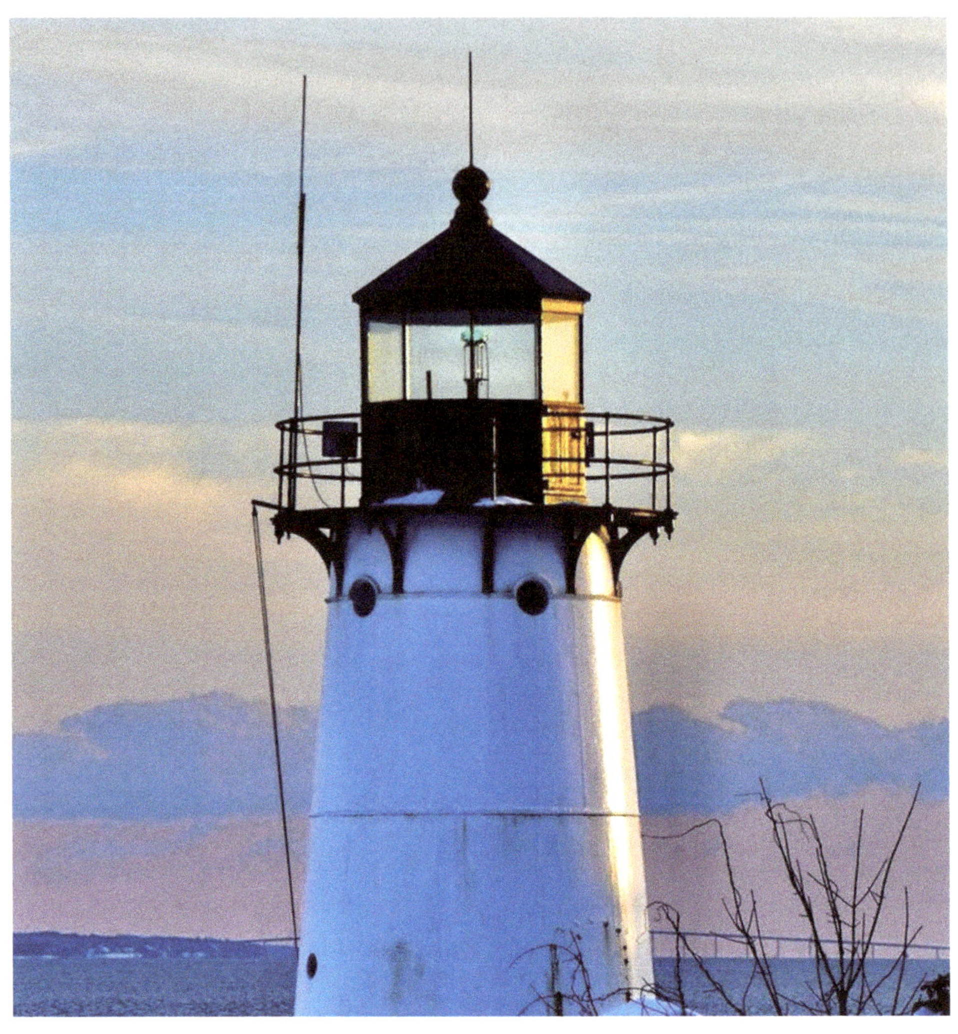

There are two ways of spreading light;
to be the candle or the mirrors that reflects it.

—Edith Wharton

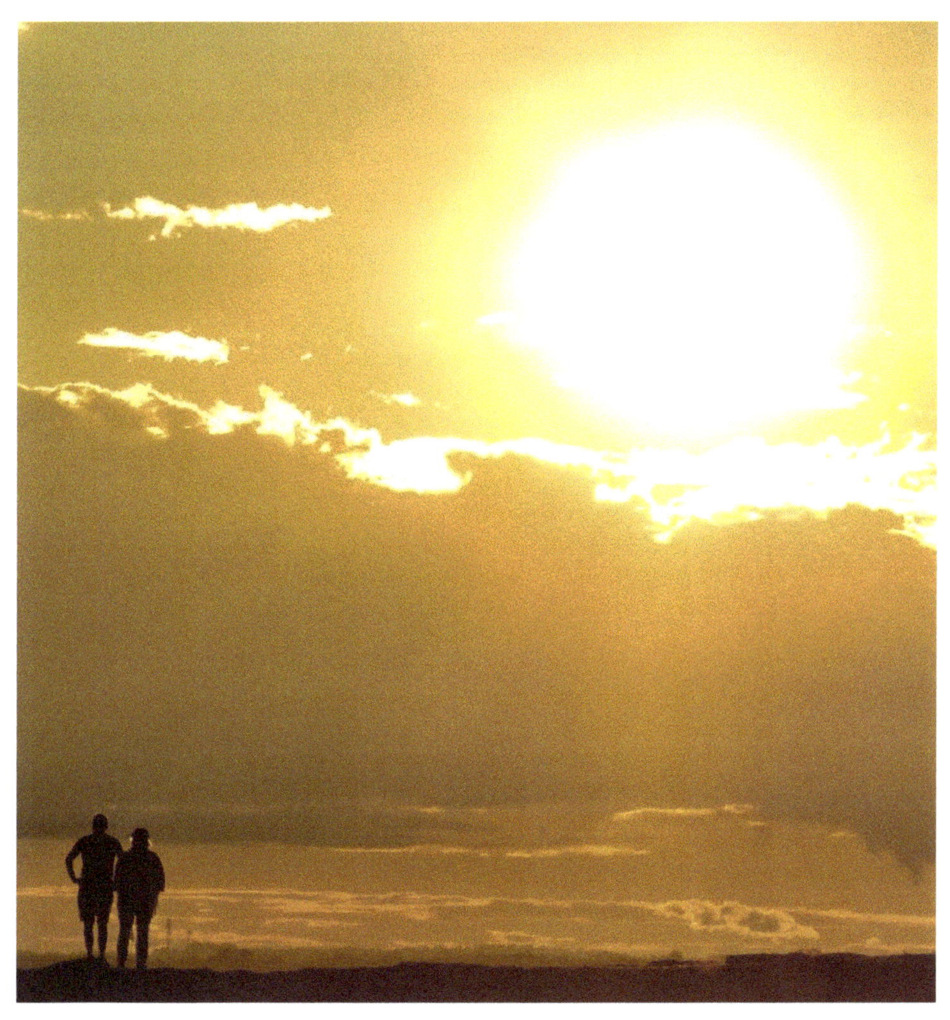

The most beautiful things in life are not things.
They are people, and places,
and memories and pictures.
They are feelings and moments
and smiles and laughter.

—Unknown

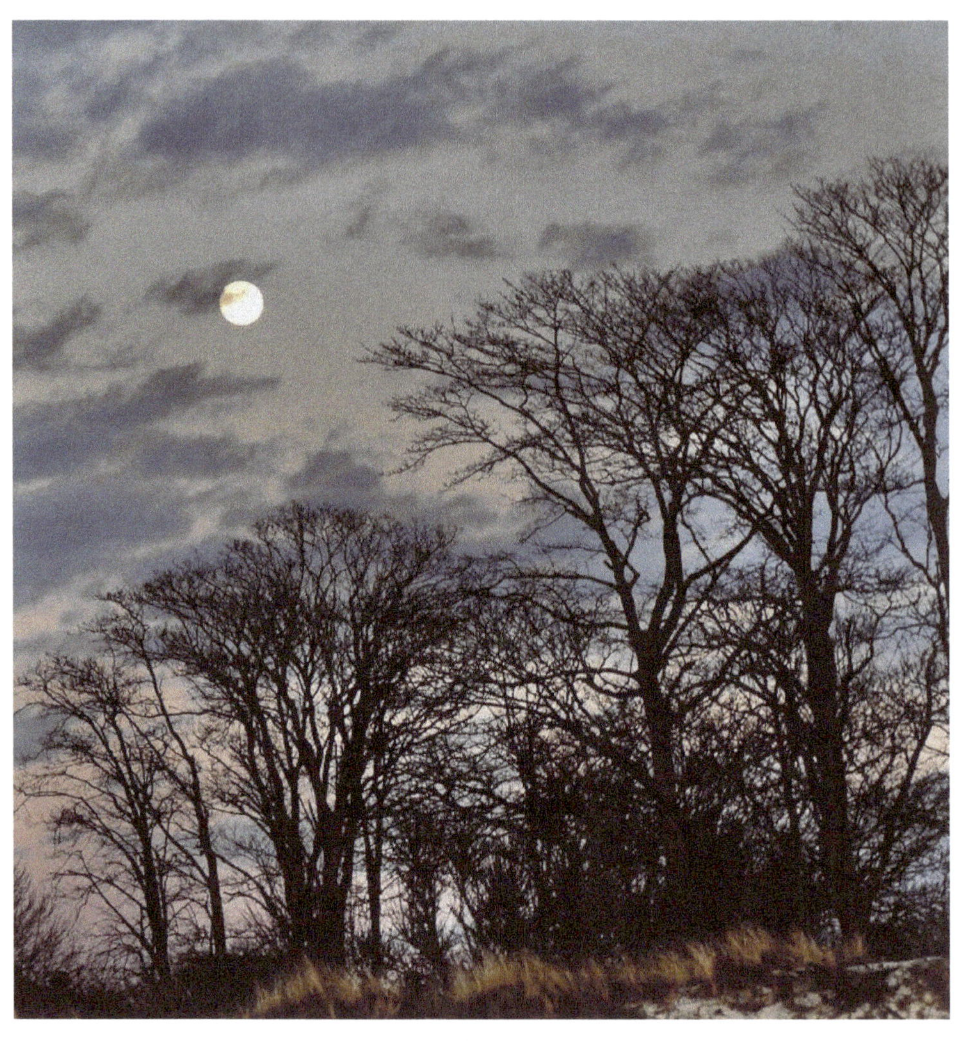

Friendship isn't a big thing,
it's a million little things.

—Becca Anderson

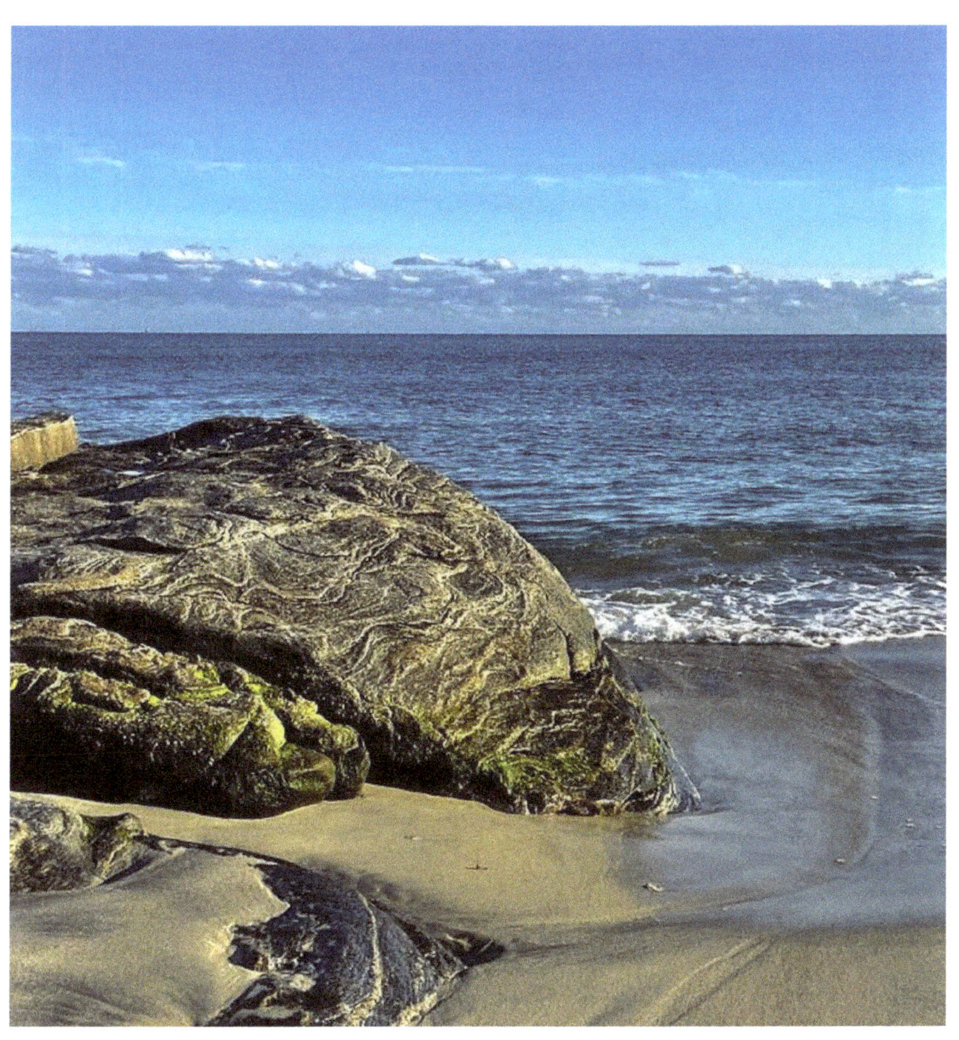

Always be willing to be inconvenienced to show up
for other people when they need you.
People are always the prize.

—Unknown

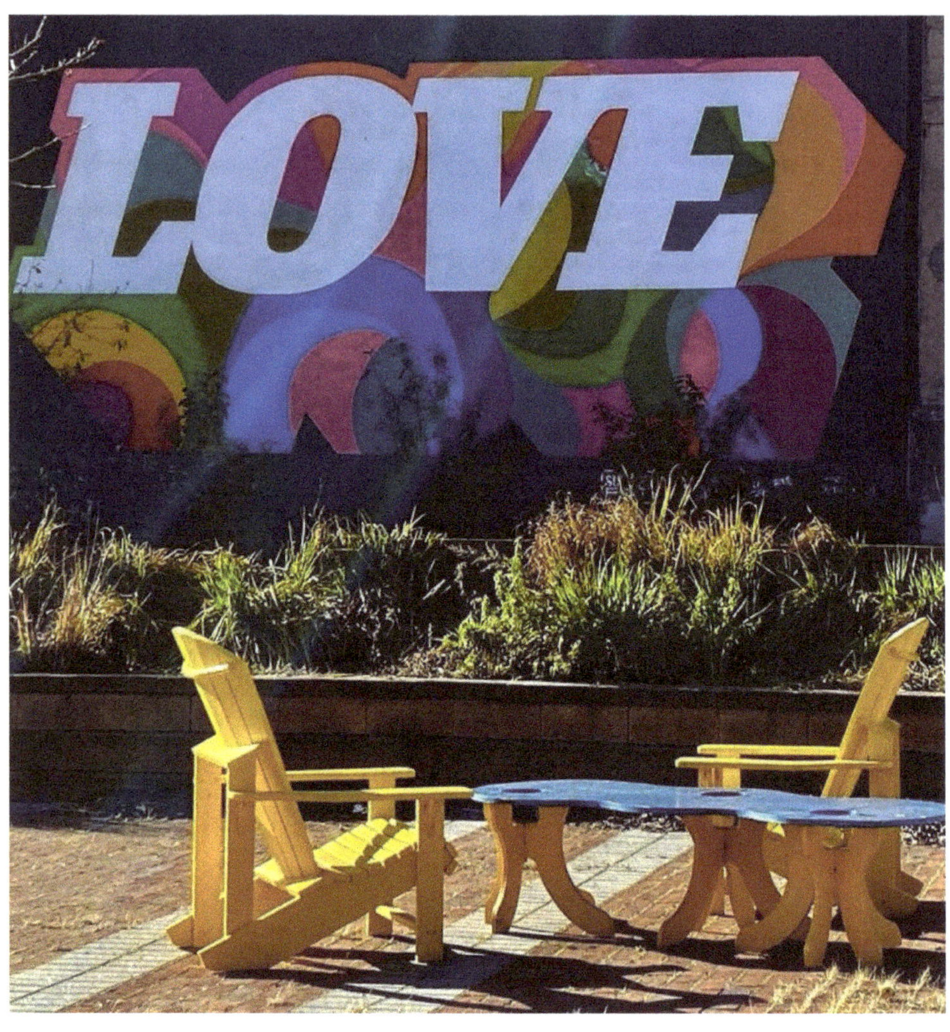

We have an empty chair at our table because
it reminds us to leave space to welcome
strangers and to always have room for love.

—Bronwyn Lea

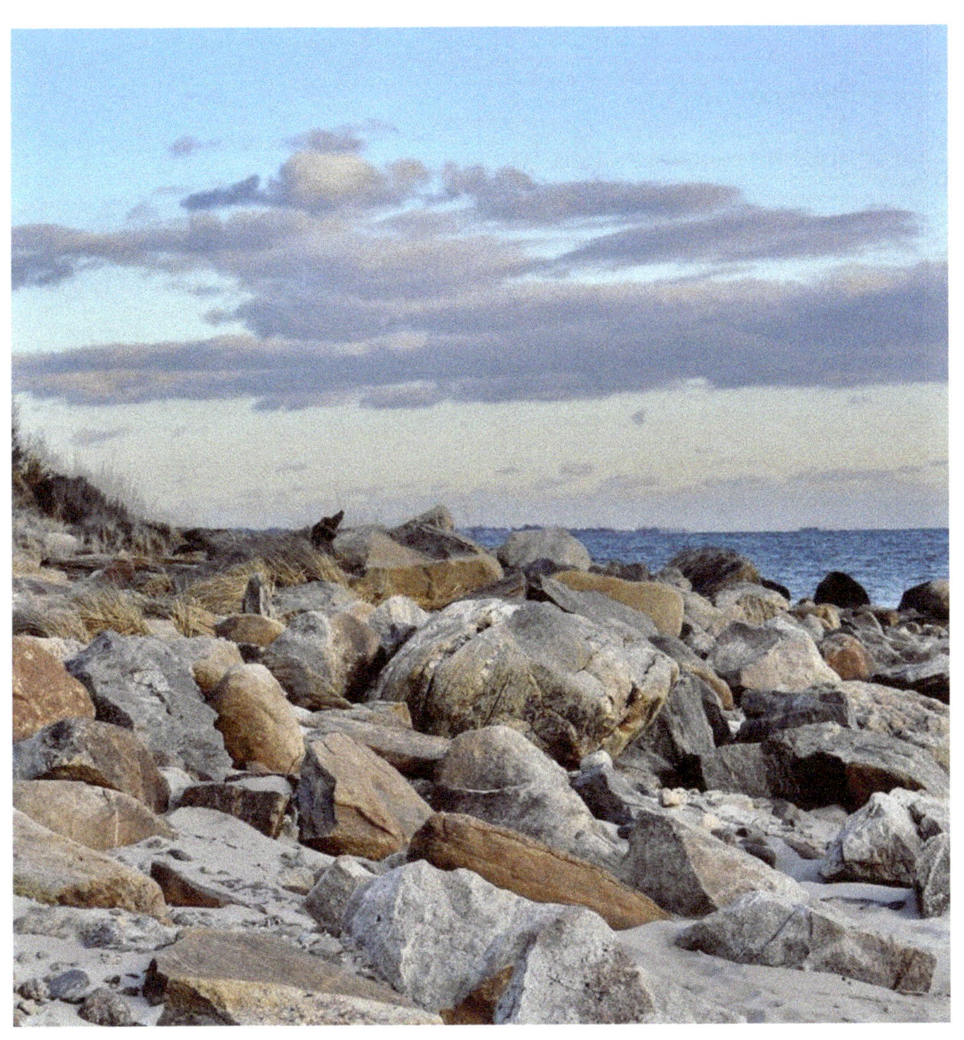

Real isn't who's with you at your celebration...
Real is who's standing next to you at rock bottom.

—Unknown

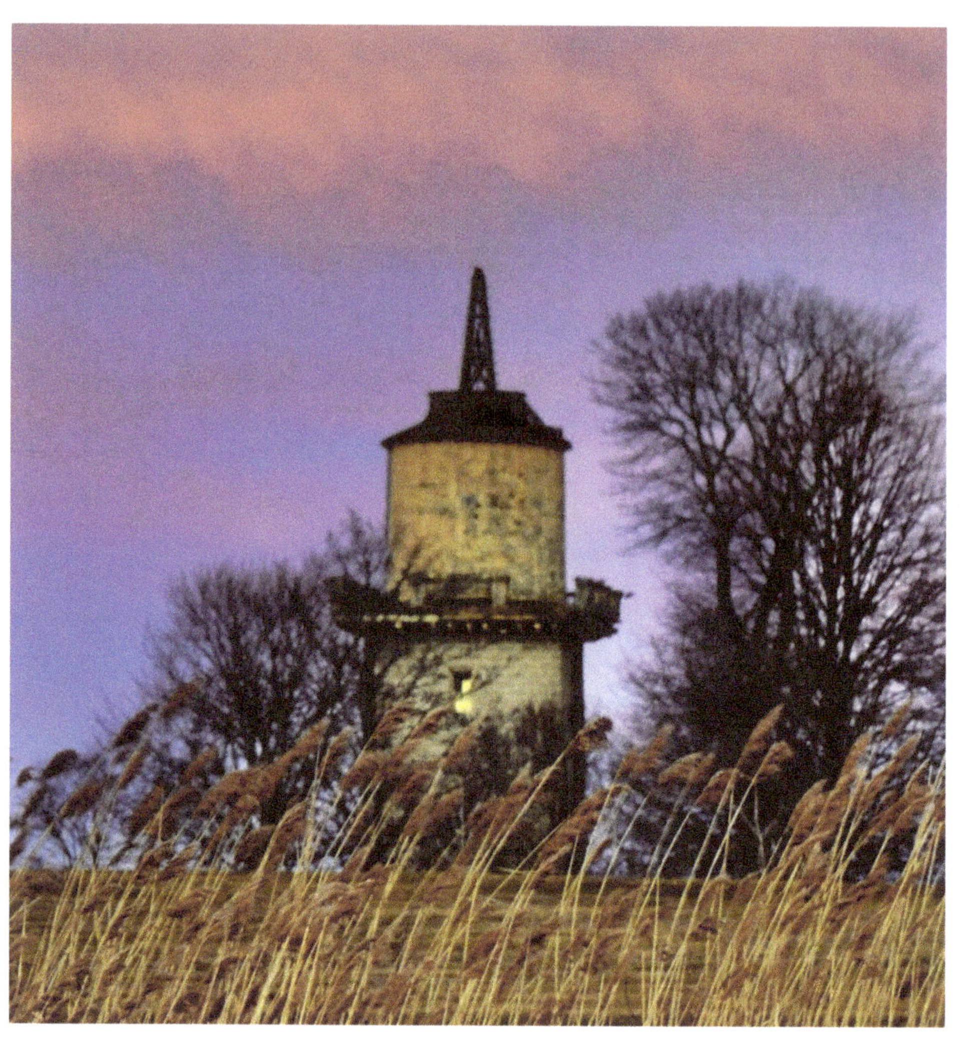

Instead of building castles against your enemies,
build bridges for them to come to you!

—Mehmet Murat ildan

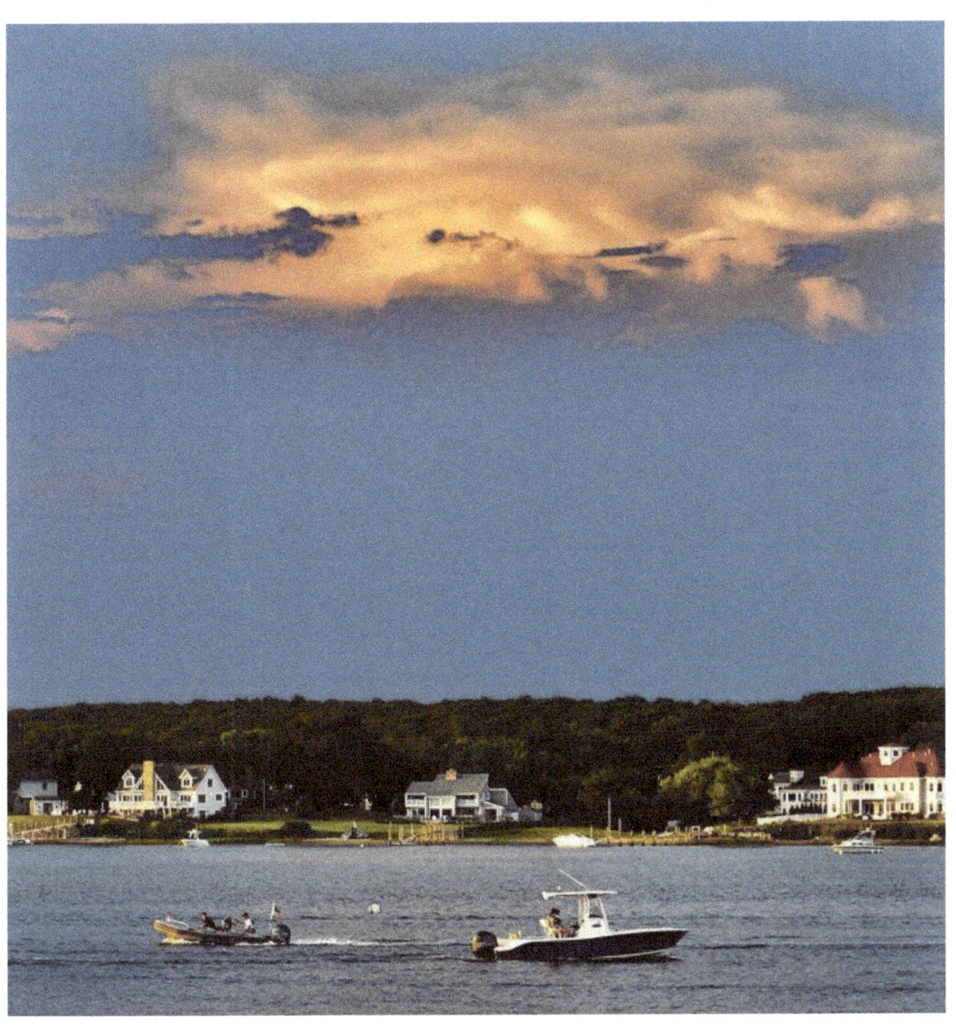

We all take different paths in life,
but no matter where we go,
we take a little of each other everywhere.

—Tim McGraw

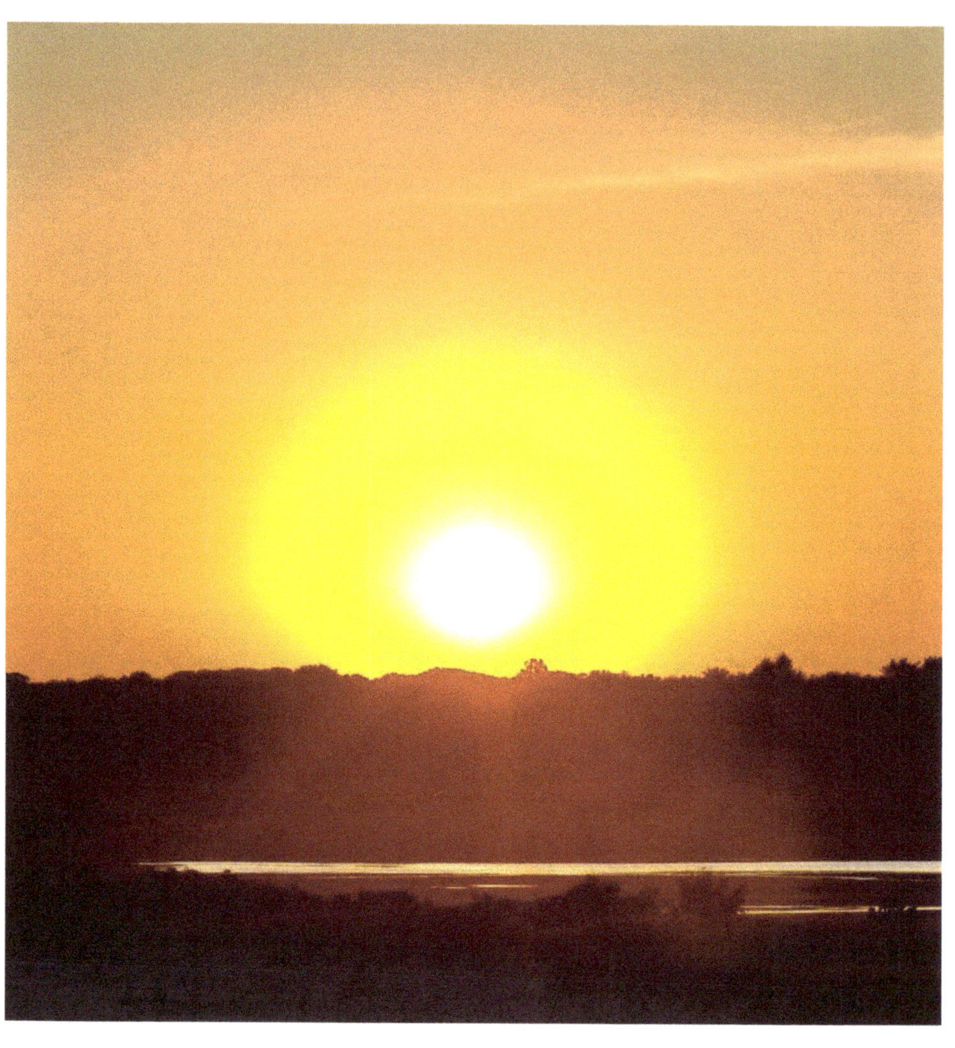

Let your light shine so brightly that others
can see their way out of the dark.

—Katrina Mayer

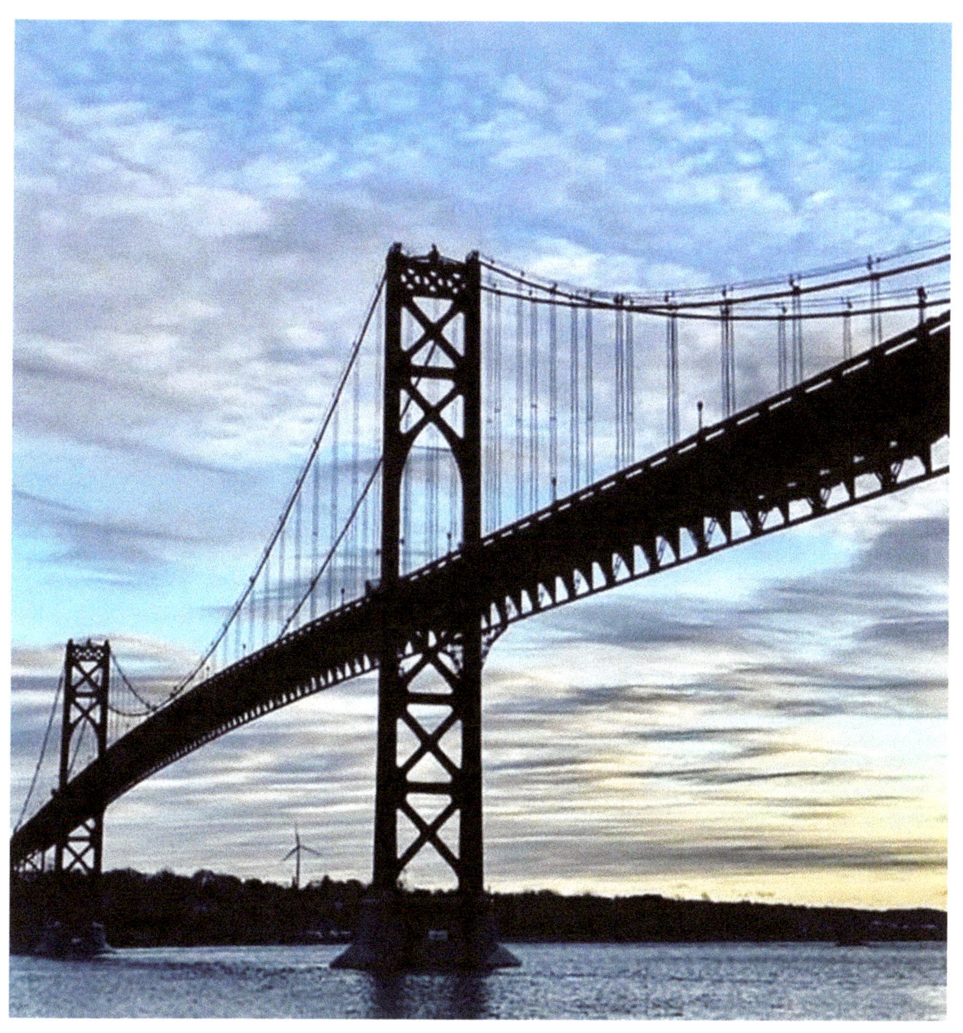

We build too many walls
and not enough bridges.

—Isaac Newton

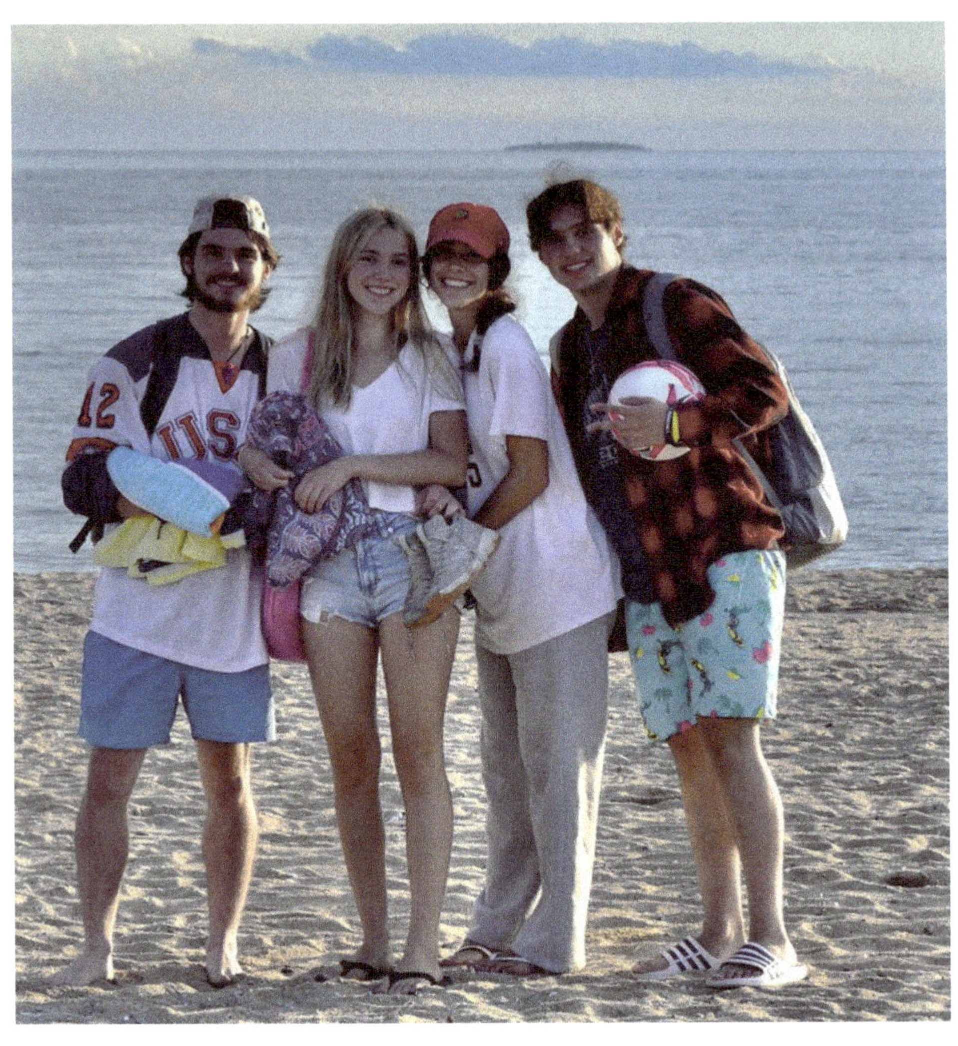

There are friends, there is family,
and then there are friends that become family.

—Jay Shetty

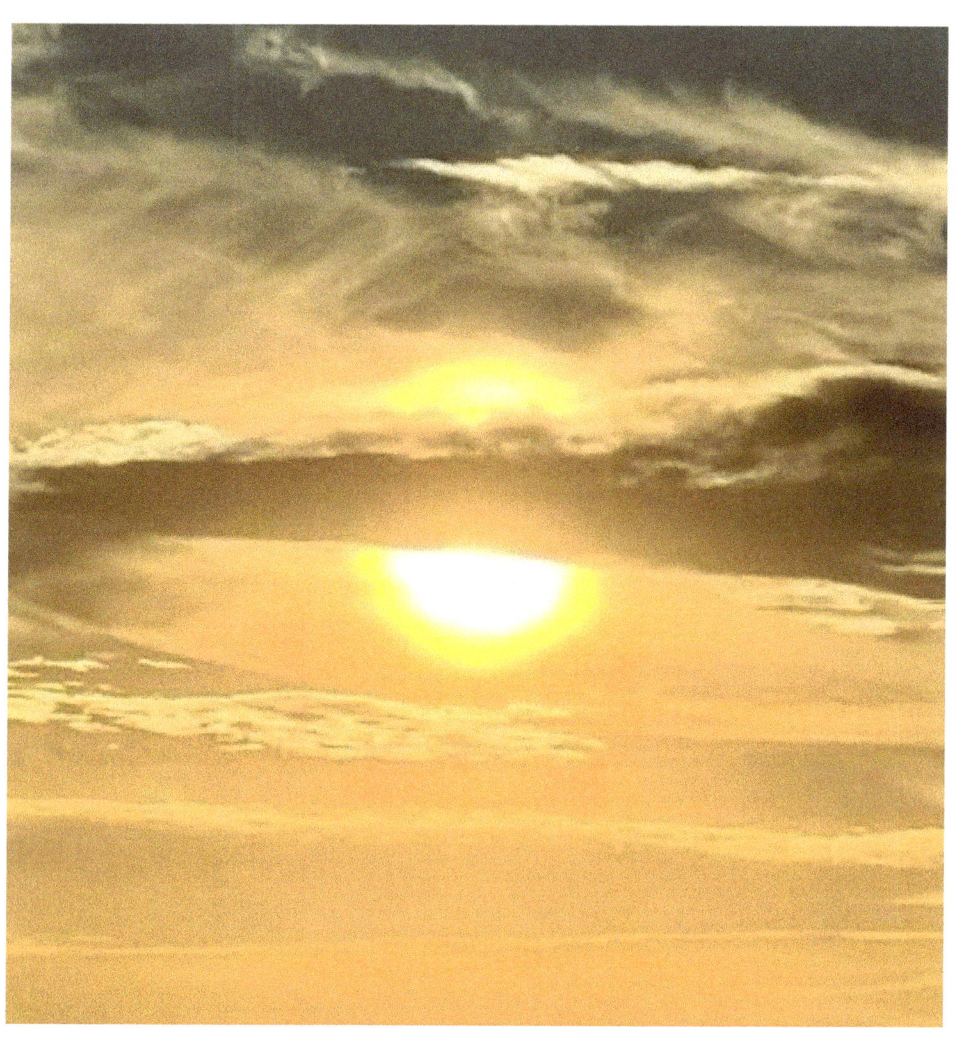

It is important in life
to be a giver and not a taker.

—Steven Fields

CHAPTER 11

Unlocking the Heart

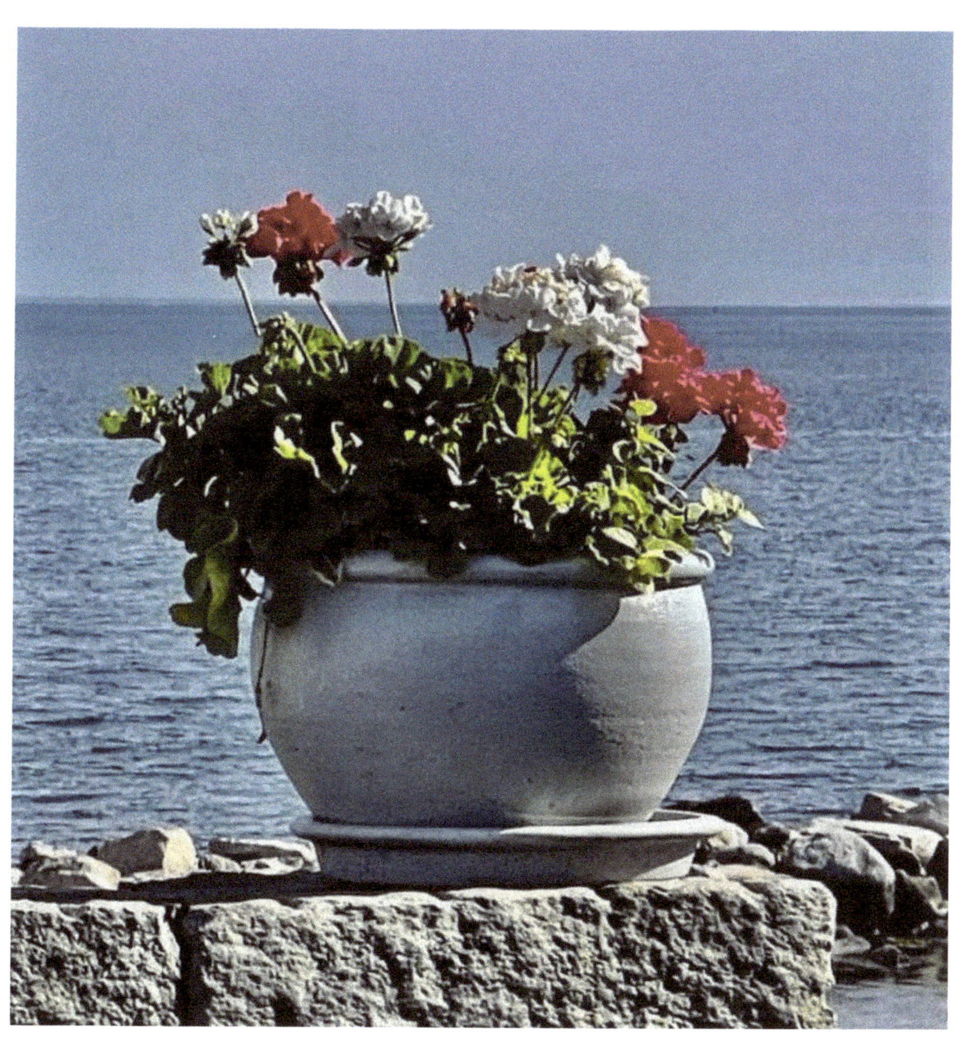

Plant your dreams in love, not fear,
and water each day with hope, not tears.

—Unknown

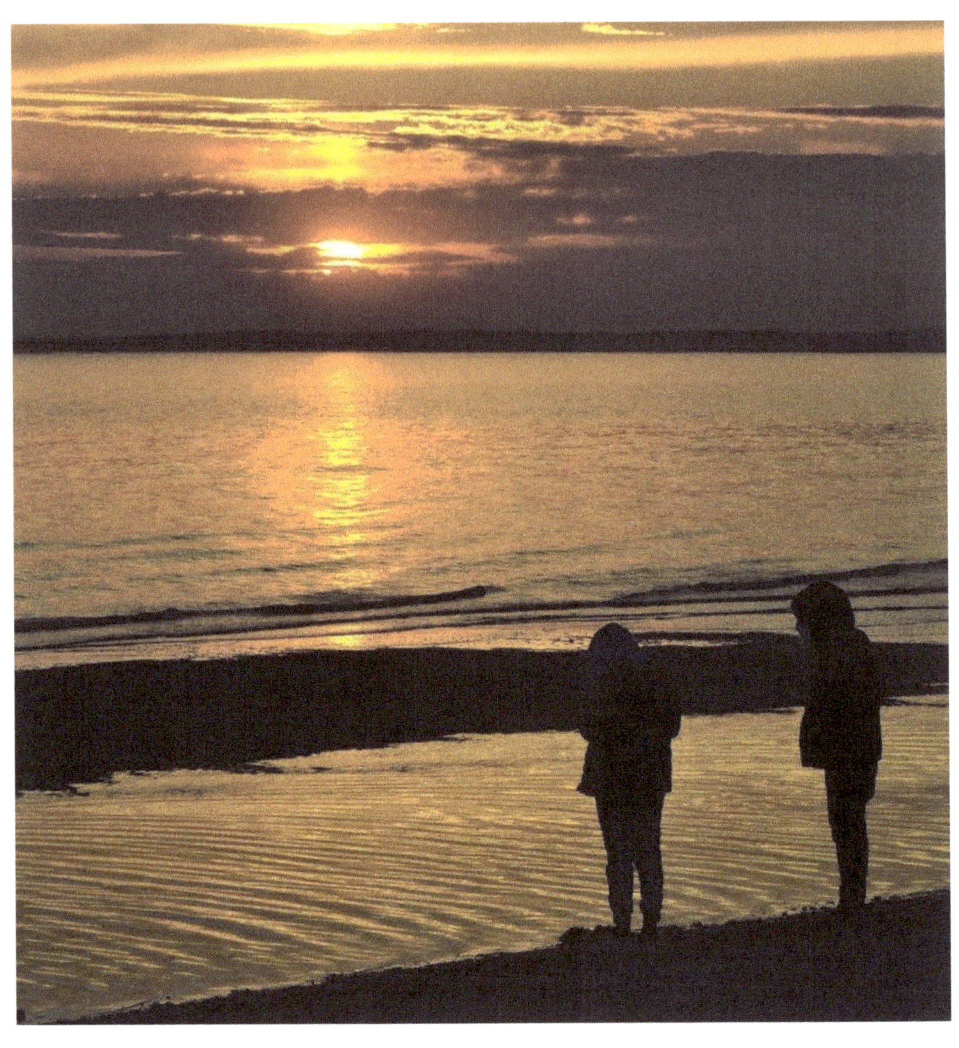

Someday you will find the one
who will watch every sunrise with you
until the sunset of your life.

—Unknown

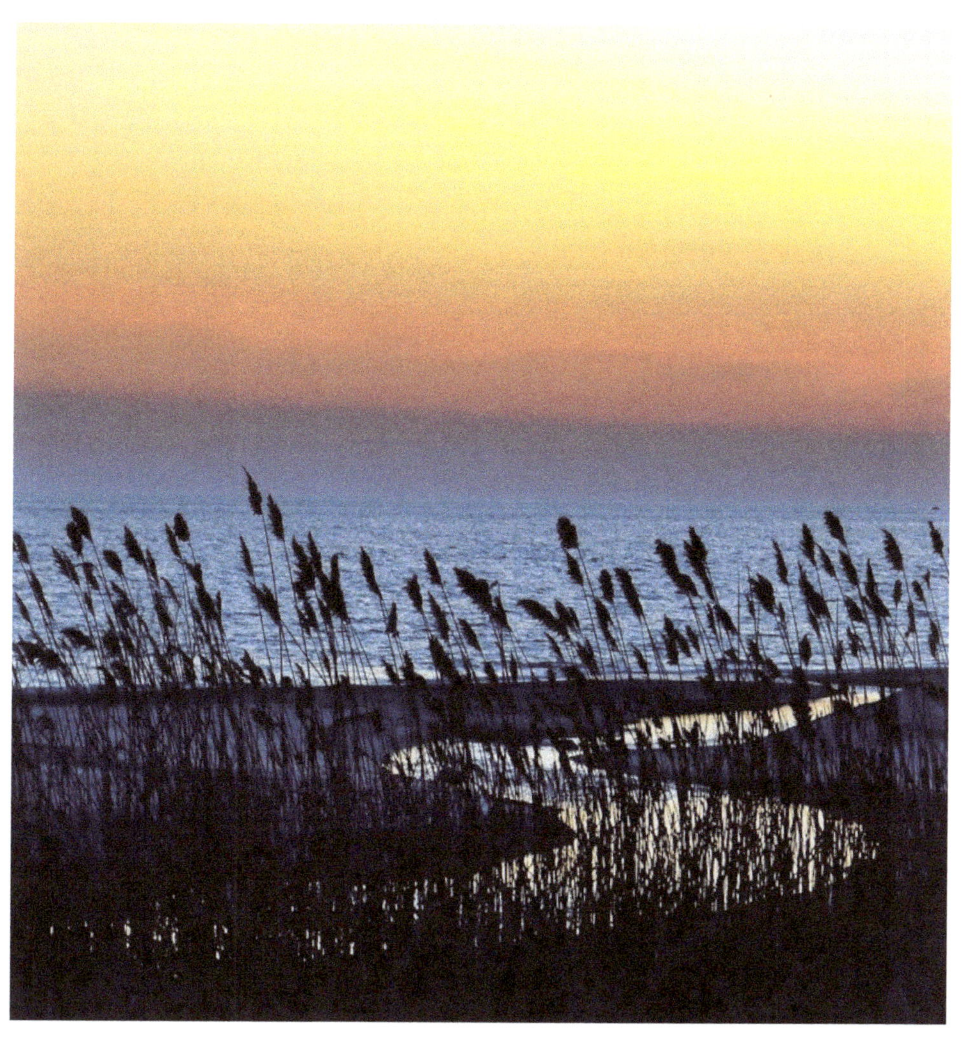

No matter who you are,
no matter where you come from,
you are beautiful.

—Michelle Obama

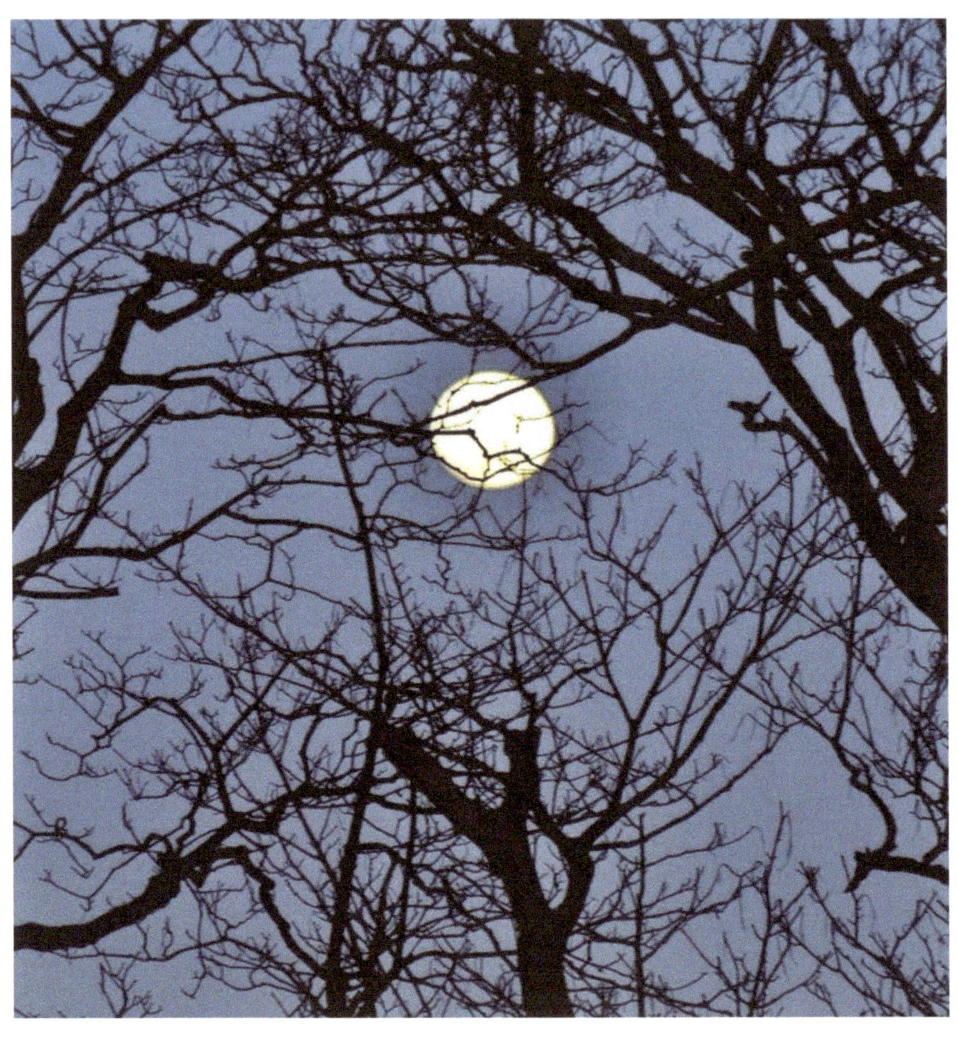

I always look up at the moon
and see it as the single most romantic
place within the cosmos.

—Tom Hanks

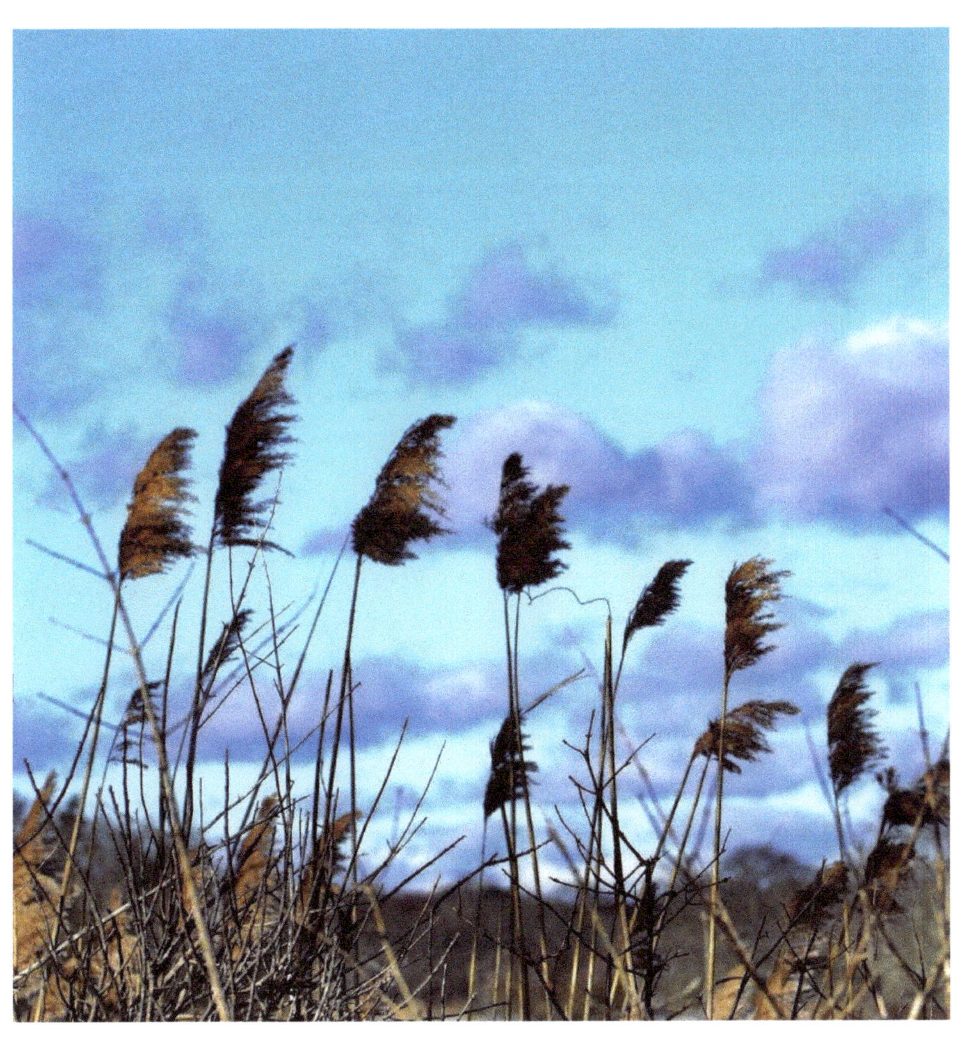

We can't do this thing
called peace and happiness
without each other.

—David Soul

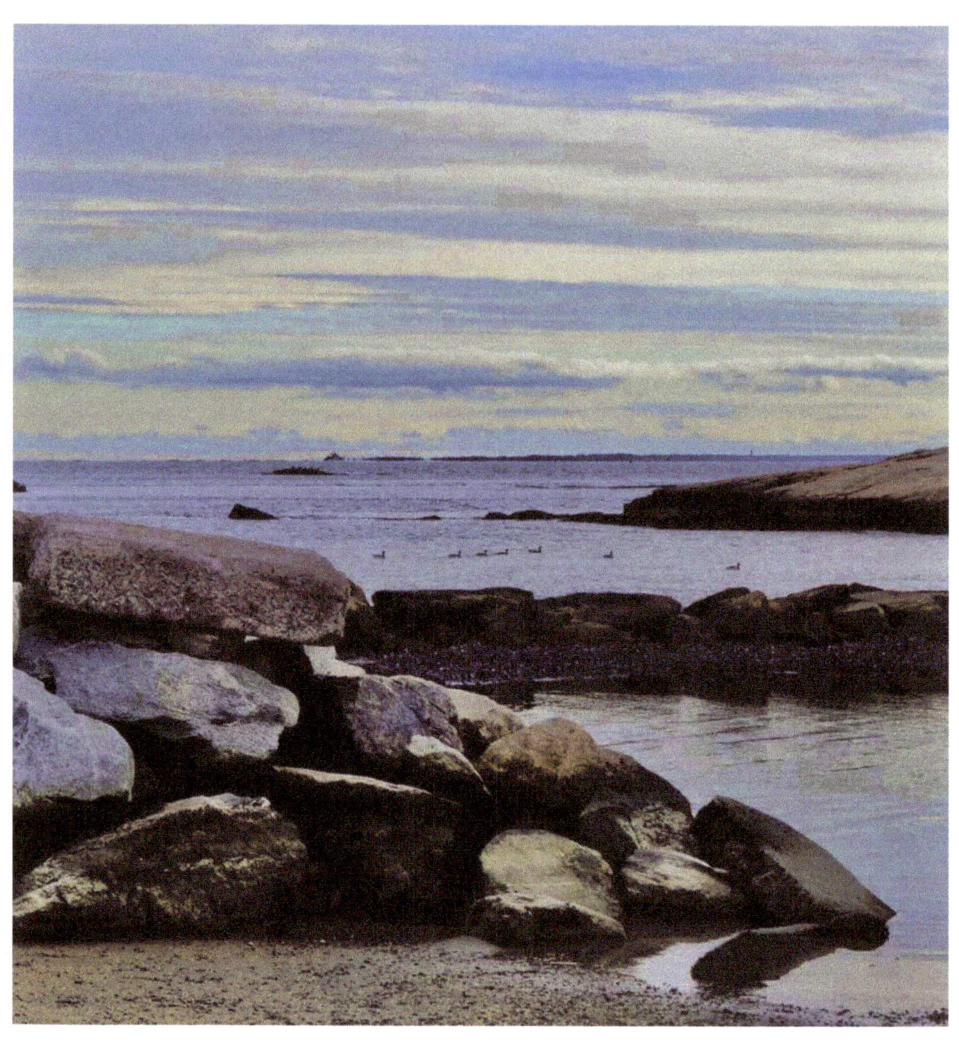

Love one another, but make not a bond of love:
Let it rather be a moving sea
between the shores of your souls.

—Kahlil Gibran

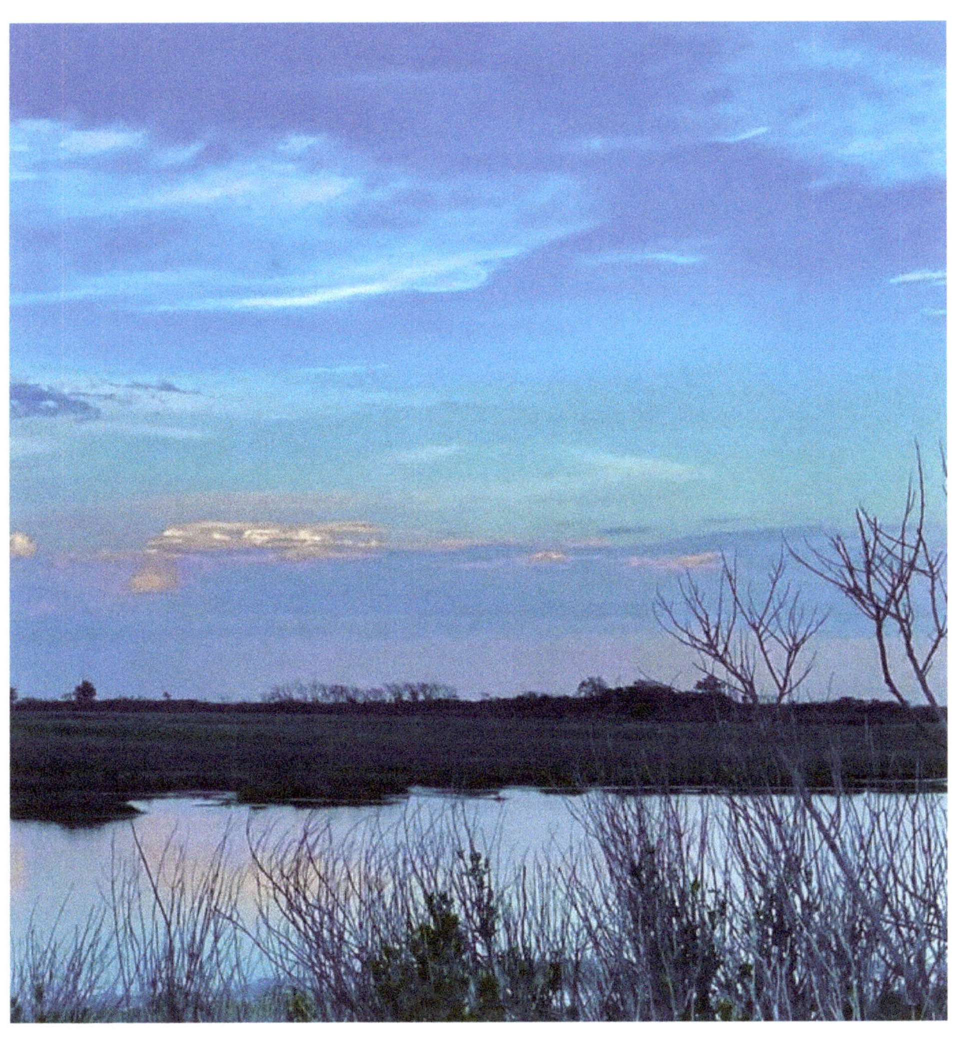

Don't be pushed around by the fears in your mind.
Be led by the dreams in your heart.

—Roy T. Bennett

CHAPTER 12

Finding Peace Within

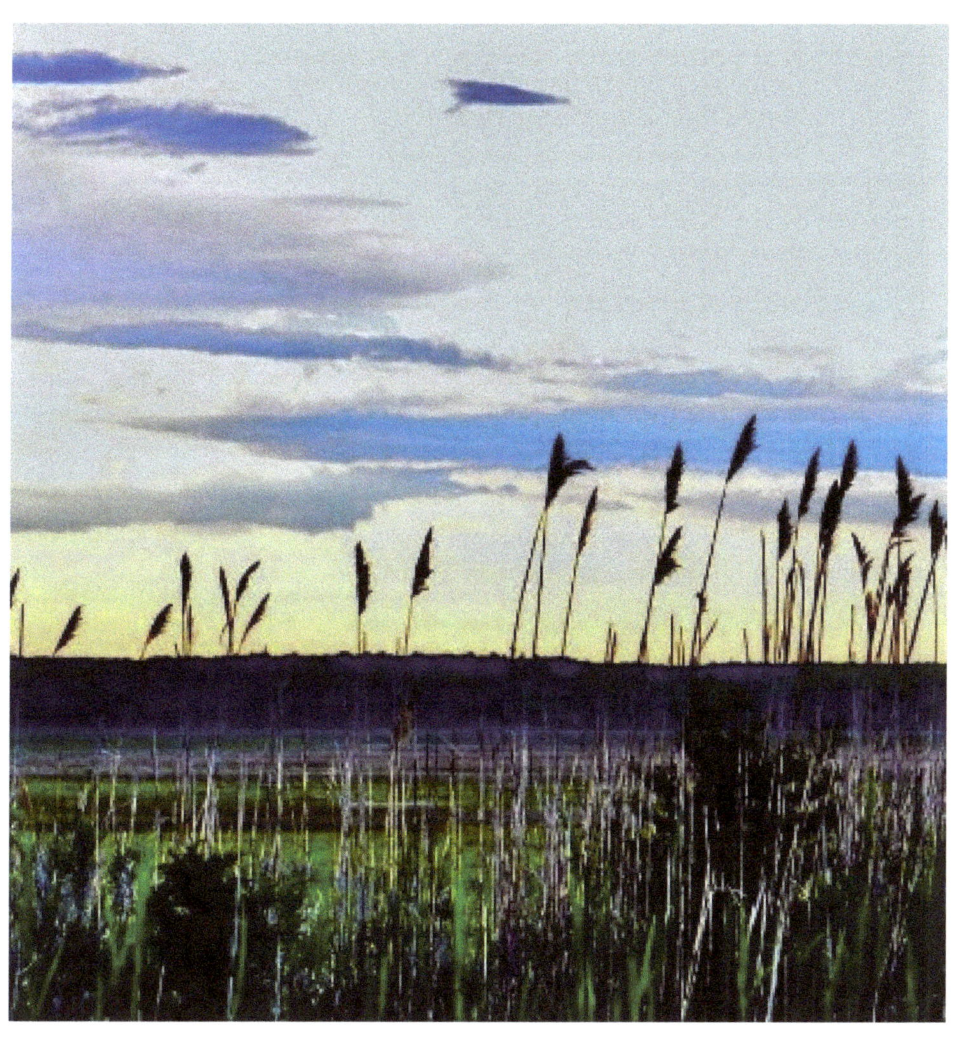

Happiness is a function of accepting what is.

—Werner Erhard

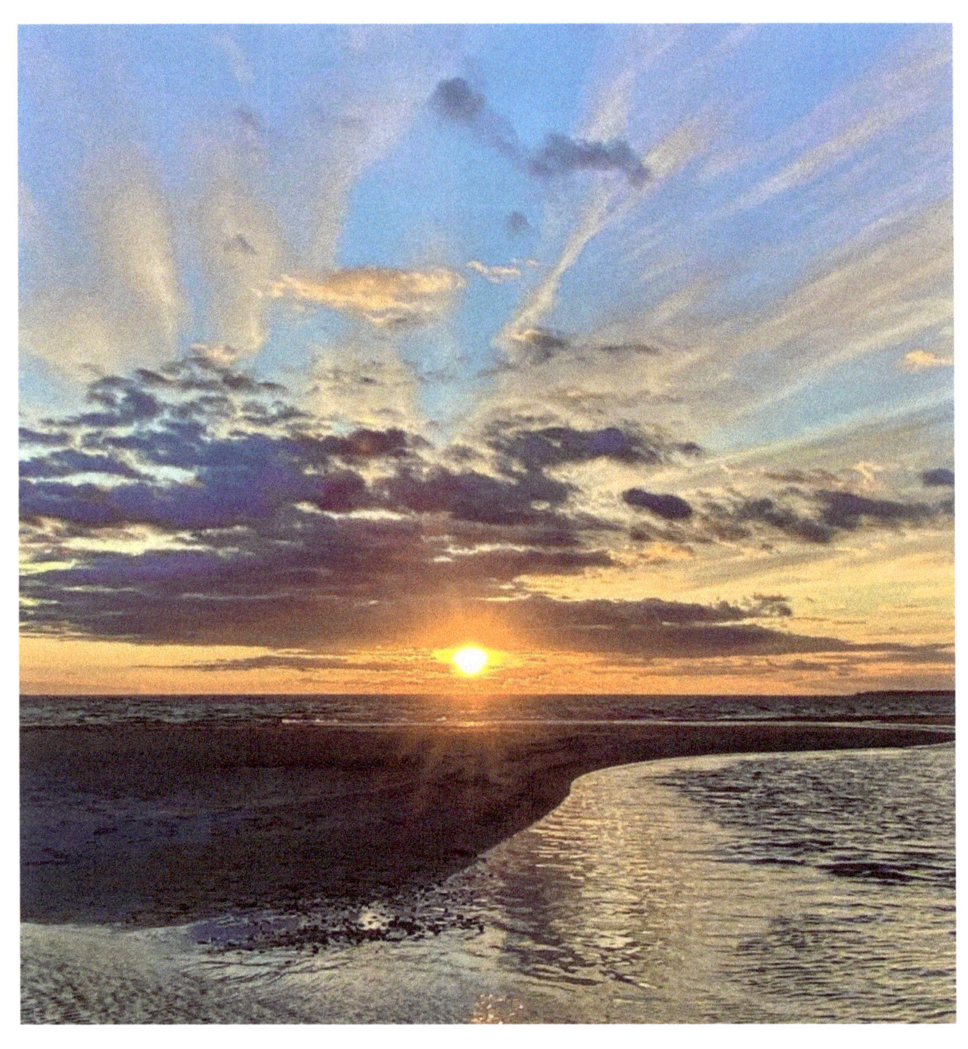

A day at the beach restores the soul.

—Unknown

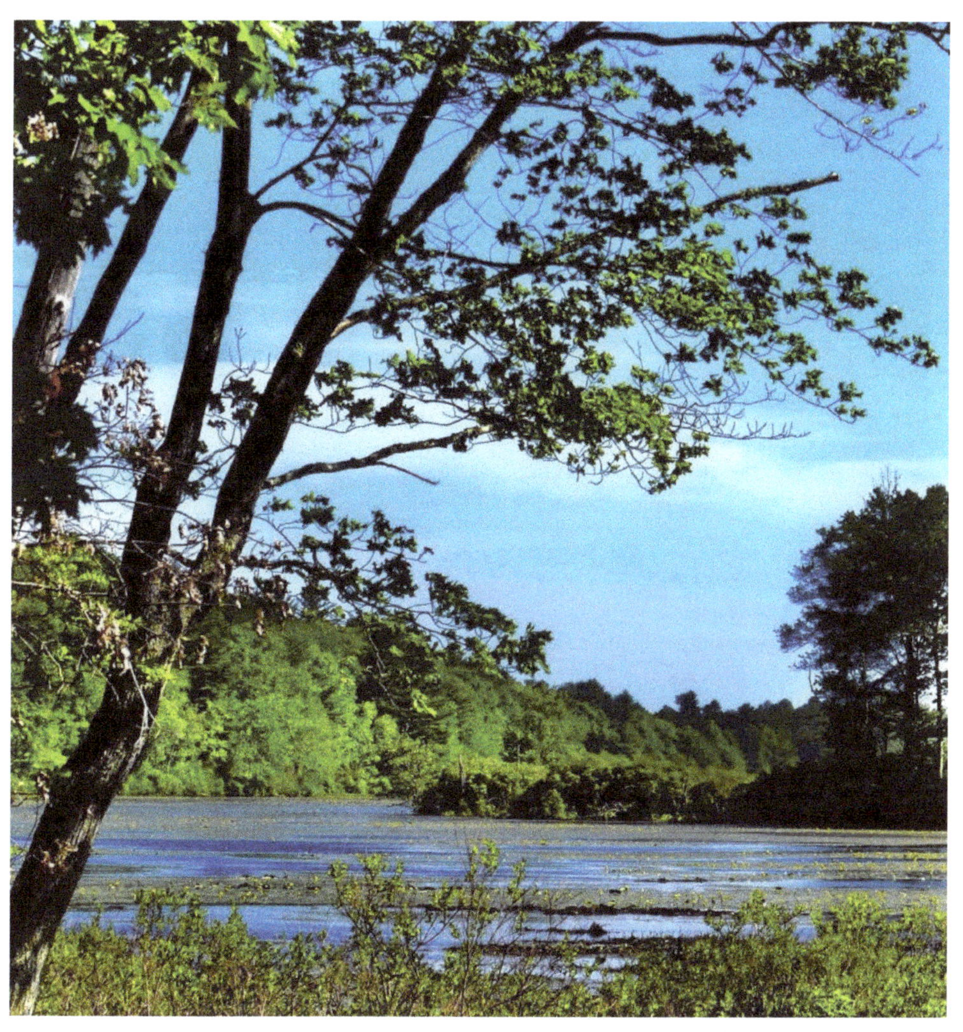

Eventually all things fall into place.
Until then, laugh at the confusion,
live for the moment, and know that
everything happens for a reason.

—Albert Schweitzer

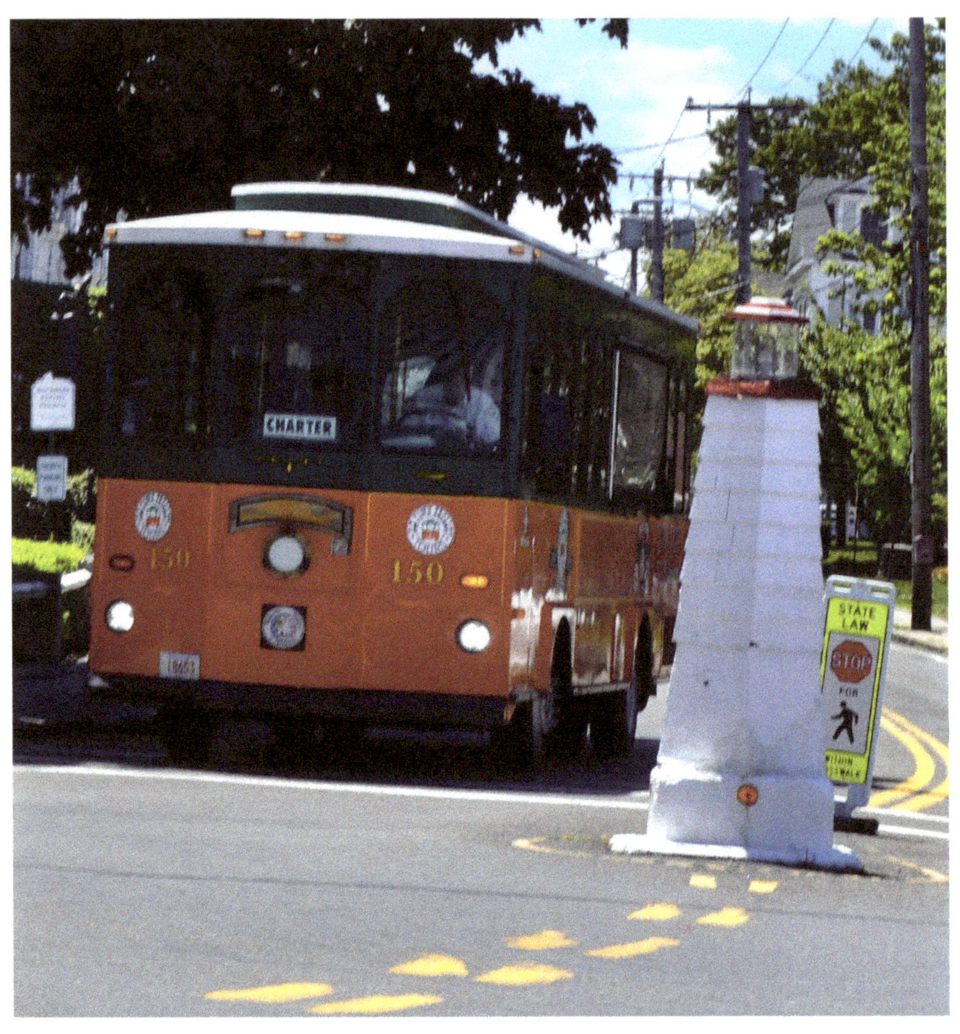

Remember that happiness is a way of travel,
not a destination.

—Roy Goodman

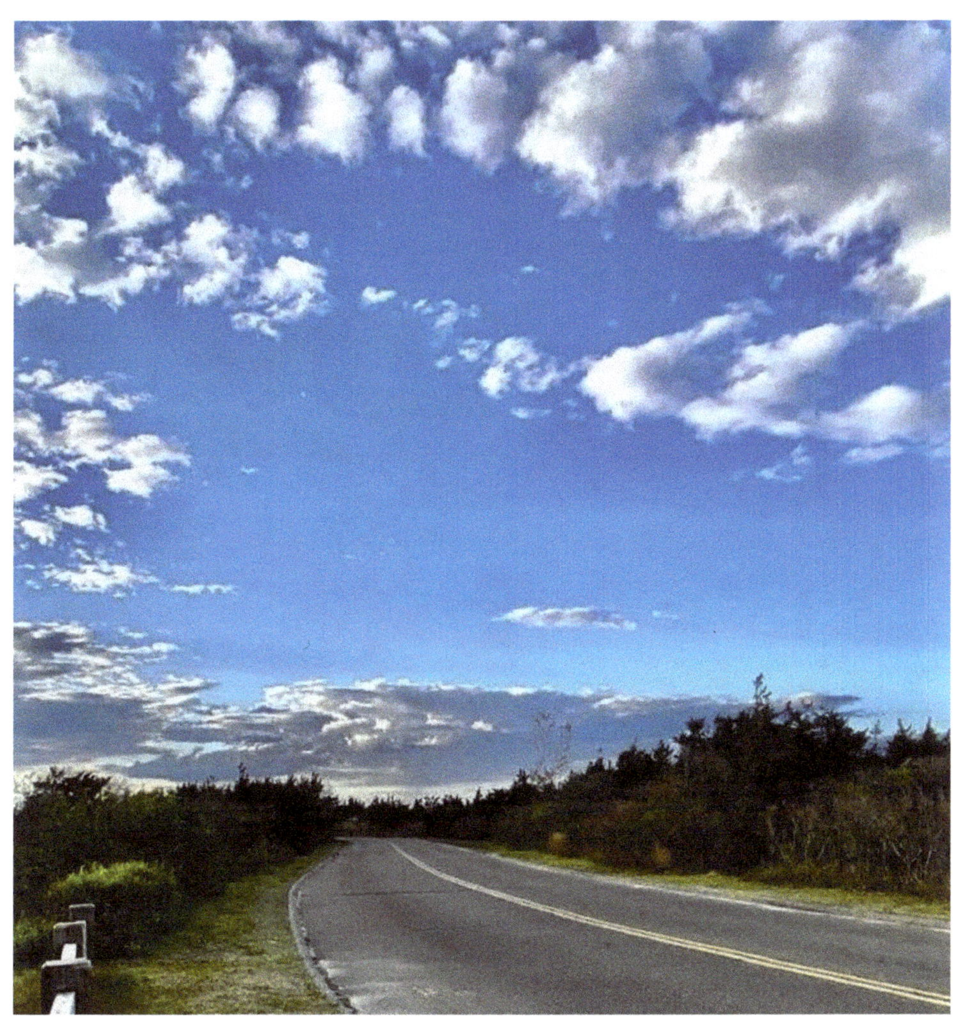

The open road still softly calls,
like a nearly forgotten song of childhood.

—Carl Sagan

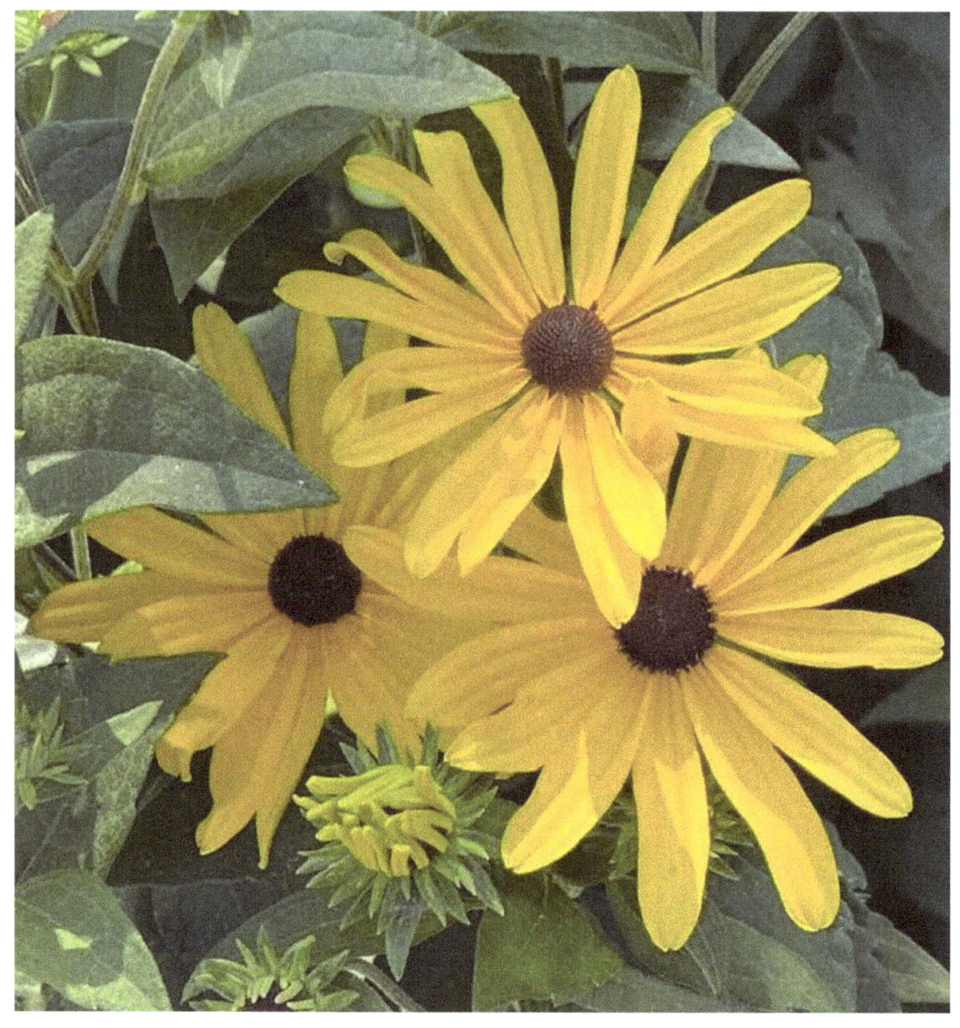

Have a mind that is open to everything
and attached to nothing.

—Dr. Wayne W. Dyer

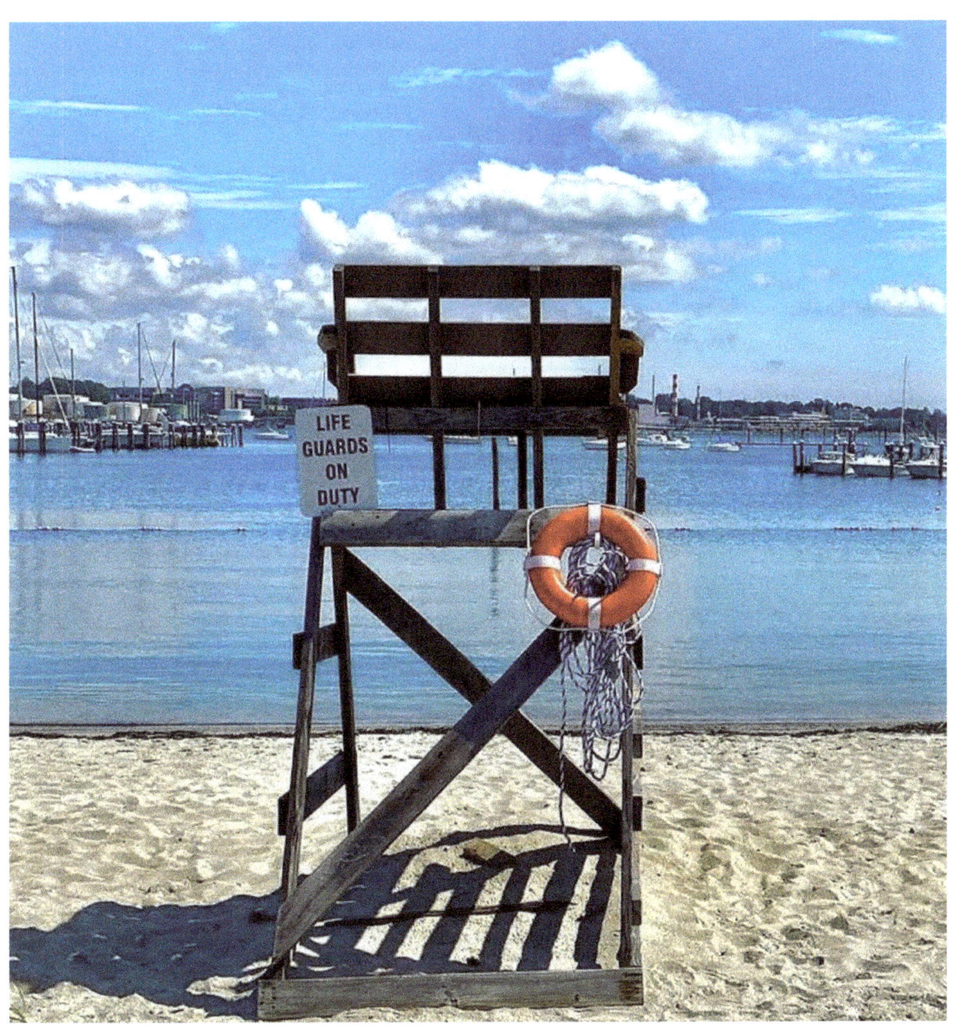

There is no duty we so much underrate
as the duty of being happy.

—Robert Louis Stevenson

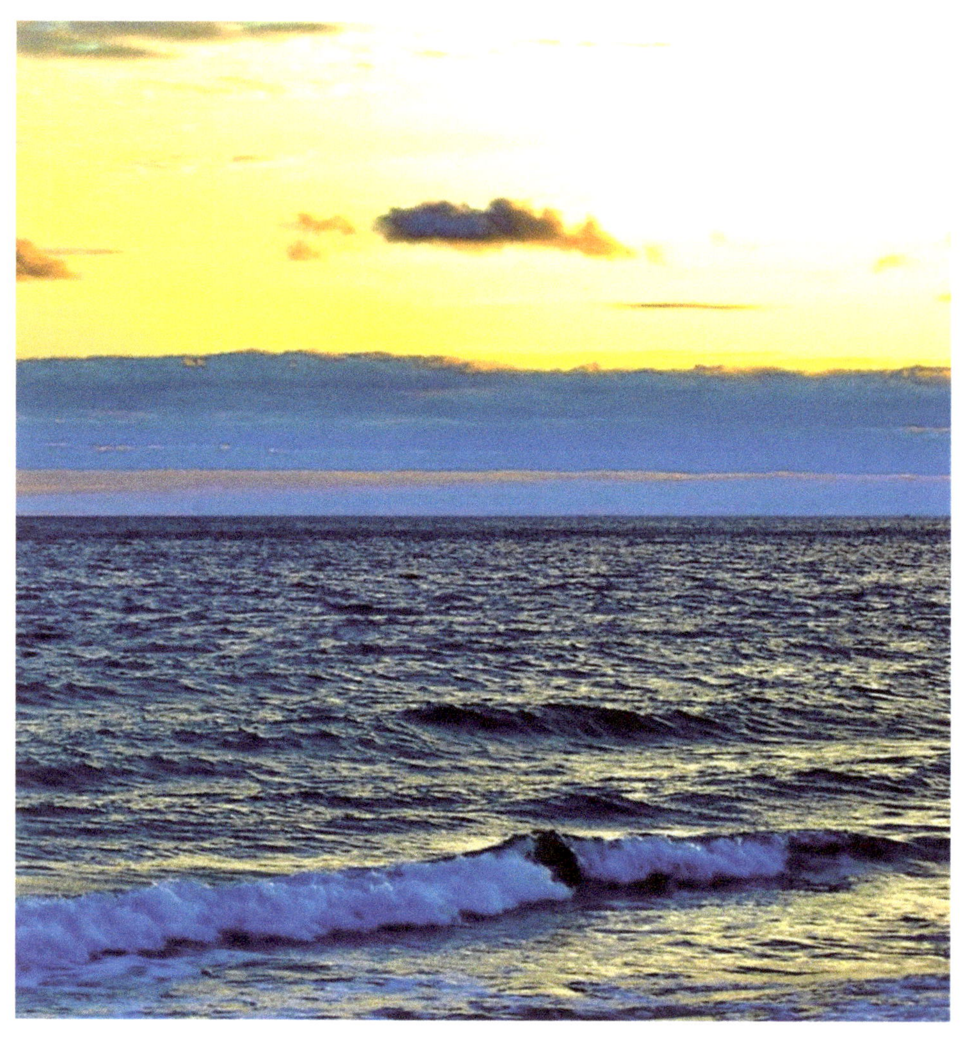

Sunsets are just little glimpses
of the golden streets of heaven.

—Unknown

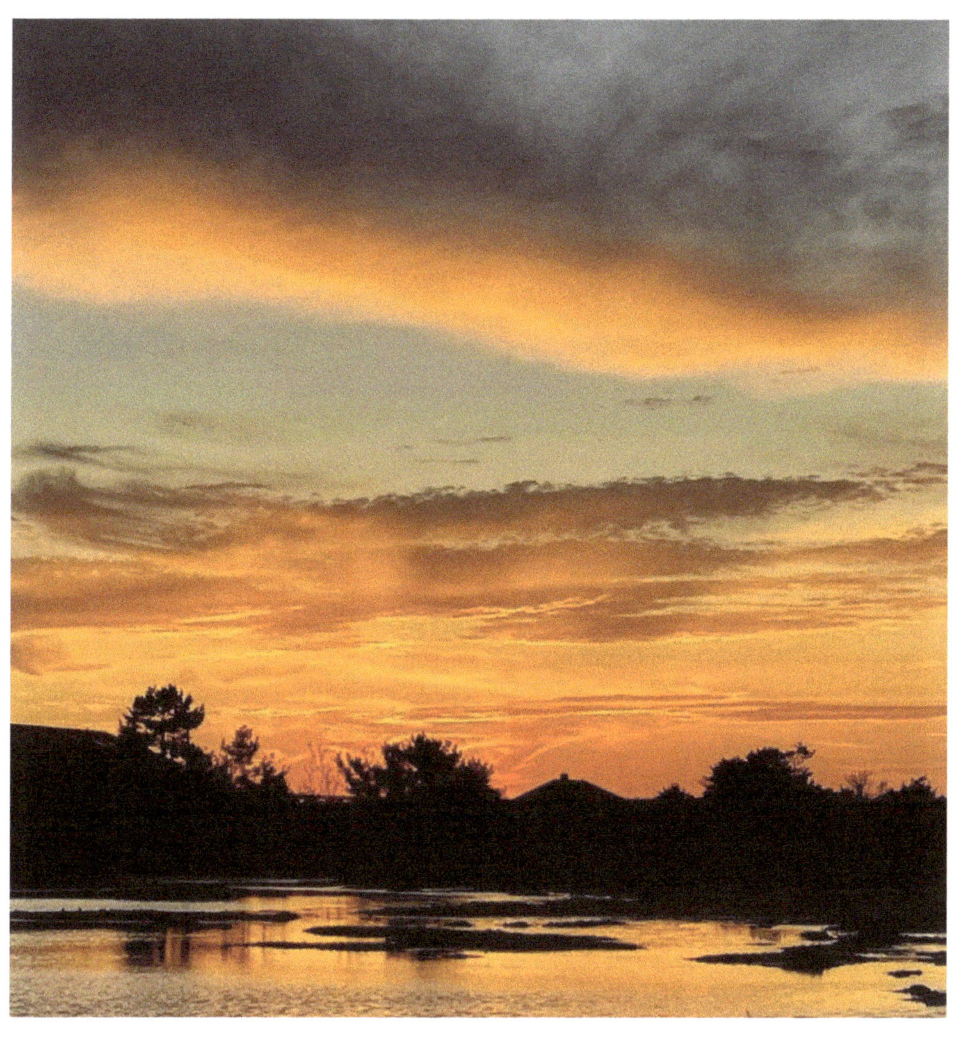

The sky takes on shades of orange during sunrise
and sunset. The color that gives you hope,
that the sun will set, only to rise again.

—Ram Charan

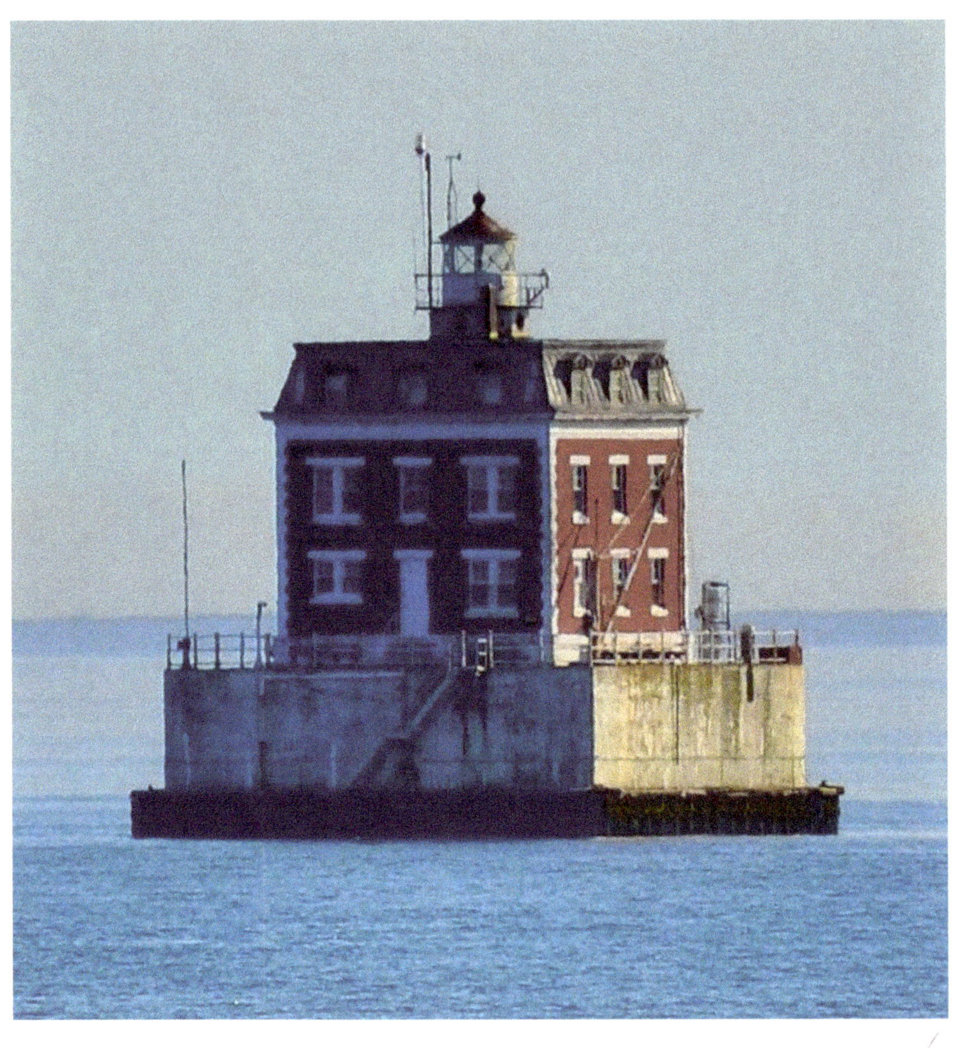

Let your light shine as an inspiration and
BE THE REASON someone believes
in the goodness of people.

—Germany Kent

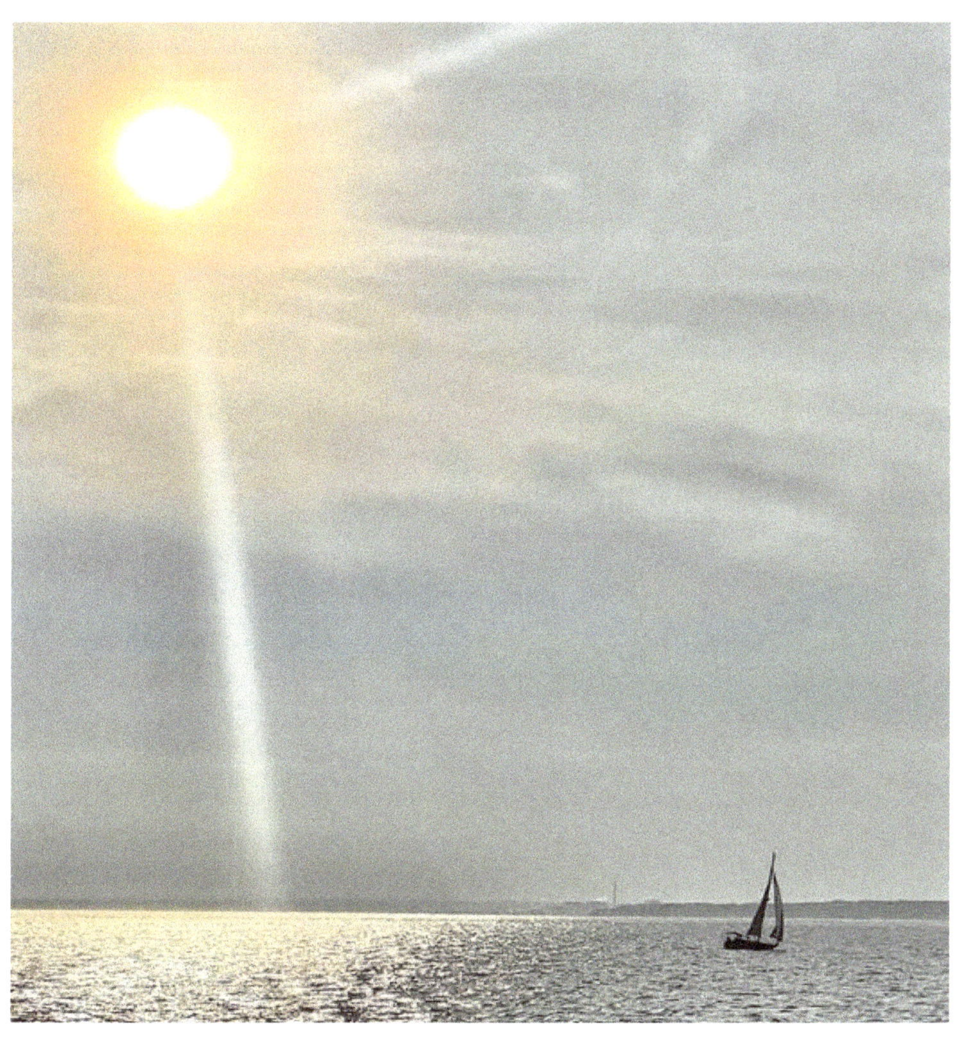

Live in the sunshine, swim in the sea,
drink the wild air.

—Ralph Waldo Emerson

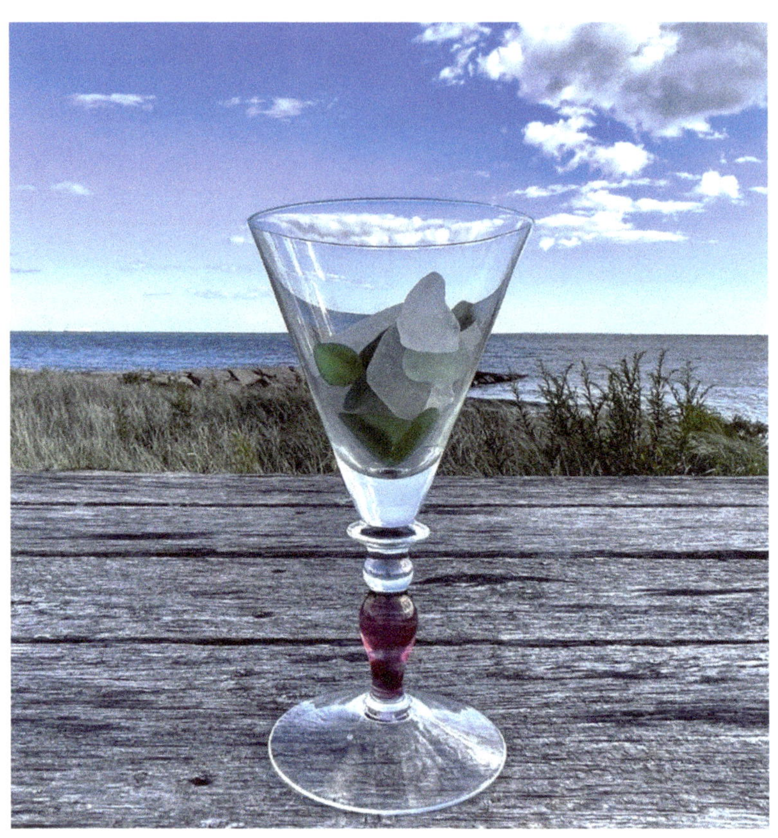

I Want to Age Like Sea Glass

I want to age like sea glass. Smoothed by tides, not broken. I want the currents of life to toss me around, shake me up and leave me feeling washed clean. I want my hard edges to soften as the years pass—made not weak but supple. I want to ride the waves, go with the flow, feel the impact of the surging tides rolling in and out.

When I am thrown against the shore and caught between the rocks and a hard place, I want to rest there until I can find the strength to do what is next. Not stuck—just waiting, pondering, feeling what it feels like to pause. And when I am ready, I will catch a wave and let it carry me along to the next place that I am supposed to be.

I want to be picked up on occasion by an unsuspected soul and carried along—just for the connection, just for the sake of appreciation and wonder. And with each encounter, new possibilities of collaboration are presented, and new ideas are born.

I want to age like sea glass so that when people see the old woman I'll become, they'll embrace all that I am. They'll marvel at my exquisite nature, hold me gently in their hands and be awed by my well-earned patina. Neither flashy nor dull, just a perfect luster. And they'll wonder, if just for a second, what it is exactly I am made of and how I got to this very here and now. And we'll both feel lucky to be in that perfectly right place at that profoundly right time.

I want to age like sea glass. I want to enjoy the journey and let my preciousness be, not in spite of the impacts of life, but because of them.

—Bernadette Noll

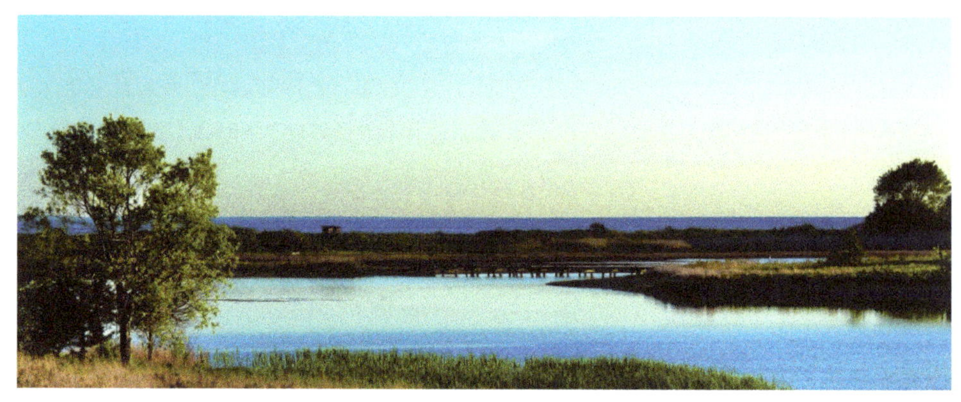

Desiderata

Go placidly amid the noise and the haste,
and remember what peace there may be in silence.
As far as possible, without surrender,
be on good terms with all persons.
Speak your truth quietly and clearly;
and listen to others, even to the dull and the ignorant;
they too have their story.
Avoid loud and aggressive persons;
they are vexatious to the spirit.
If you compare yourself with others,
you may become vain or bitter,
for always there will be greater
and lesser persons than yourself.
Enjoy your achievements as well as your plans.
Keep interested in your own career,
however humble; it is a real possession in the changing
fortunes of time.
Exercise caution in your business affairs,
for the world is full of trickery.
But let this not blind you to what virtue there is;
many persons strive for high ideals,
and everywhere life is full of heroism.
Be yourself. Especially do not feign affection.

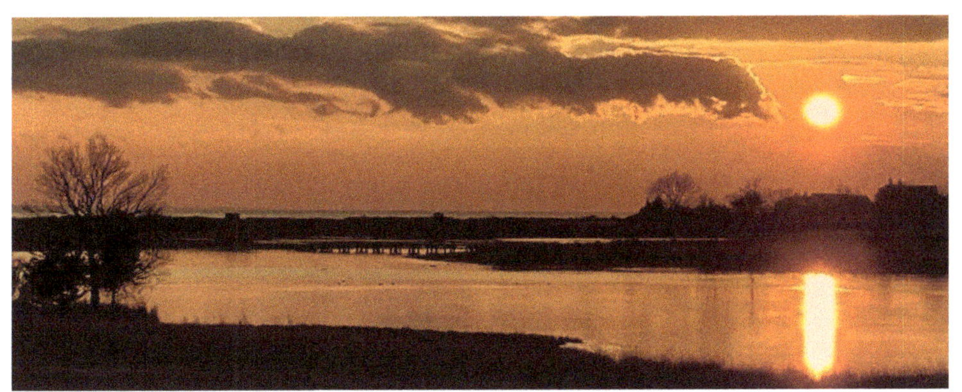

Neither be cynical about love,
for in the face of all aridity and disenchantment,
it is as perennial as the grass.
Take kindly the counsel of the years,
gracefully surrendering the things of youth.
Nurture strength of spirit
to shield you in sudden misfortune.
But do not distress yourself with dark imaginings.
Many fears are born of fatigue and loneliness.
Beyond a wholesome discipline,
be gentle with yourself.
You are a child of the universe no less than the trees and
the stars; you have a right to be here.
And whether or not it is clear to you,
no doubt the universe is unfolding as it should.
Therefore be at peace with God,
whatever you conceive Him to be.
And whatever your labors and aspirations,
in the noisy confusion of life,
keep peace in your soul.
With all its sham, drudgery, and broken dreams,
it is still a beautiful world.
Be cheerful. Strive to be happy.

—Max Ehrmann

Harry Thomas' Twelve Principles For Living Your Best Life

- ❖ Peace is keeping a humble perspective by focusing on the bigger picture. It's not all about me.
- ❖ Peace is maintaining an attitude of gratitude and expressing appreciation to others where it is due.
- ❖ Peace is recognizing and embracing the strength and personal power that is within each of us.
- ❖ Peace is found through self-reflecting, which is the root to strong character.
- ❖ Peace is being courageous enough to step out of the comfort zone and seize the opportunities that life has to offer.
- ❖ Peace is finding direction and purpose and walking that path confidently.
- ❖ Peace is embracing my responsibilities with a strong work ethic.
- ❖ Peace is accepting the challenge of obstacles and creatively identifying strategies for overcoming them.
- ❖ Peace is trusting my intuition when making tough decisions, recognizing that the answer lies within me.
- ❖ Peace is nurturing positive social connections and letting go of toxic ones.
- ❖ Peace is opening your heart and being willing to be vulnerable and authentic.
- ❖ Peace is found by being one with nature. Peace is within reach down by the sea.

About the Author

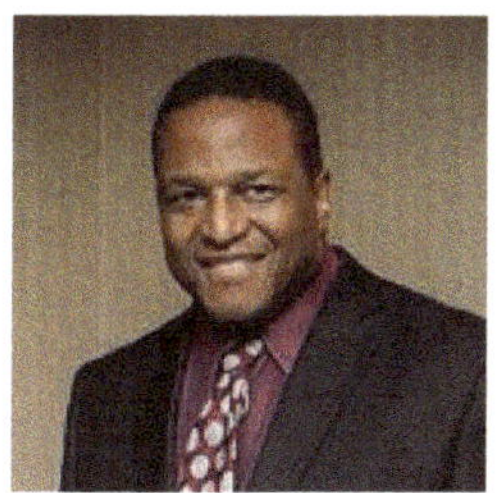

Harry L. Thomas, MSW
Author, Actor, Producer,
Adjunct Professor of Social Work

Finding Peace by the Sea is Harry Thomas' second book. In 2020, he published *Peace by the Sea: Inspiring Images and Quotes to Light Your Way.* Harry is an active humanitarian who enjoys helping people get on the right track to live their best lives. He earned his master's degree from the University of Connecticut's School of Social Work. As an adjunct professor, he presented engaging lectures at Eastern Connecticut State University. He lives for lively conversations on what really matters to people. His friends look forward to his daily social-media posts of his personal photography carefully matched with uplifting quotes.

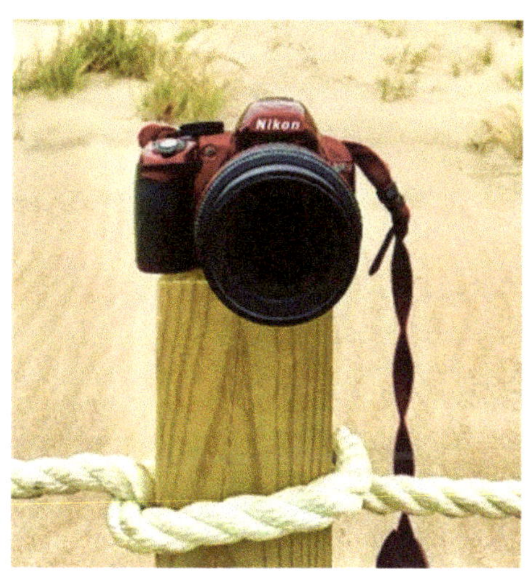

Harry is also an actor, writer, and producer. Recently, he has written and produced commercials and public-service announcements dealing with current social issues, such as social justice, mental health, and personal well-being. He thrives on inspiring change through careful combinations of images and words. Harry commonly appears as an actor in television shows, movies, and commercials. He is proud to be a member of the Screen Actors Guild – American Federation of Television and Radio Artists (SAG-AFTRA). He has appeared with Hollywood actors including Meryl Streep, Al Pacino, Kevin Costner, Adam Sandler, and others. Due to his deep love of music, he also enjoys the art of freelancing as a video DJ. He is a member of the Chamber of Commerce of Eastern Connecticut and the Greater Norwich Chamber of Commerce.

Photography has captivated Harry ever since receiving his first camera as a child. Capturing appealing moments and visual images on film has always been a passion. He has earned local recognition and awards for his photography throughout his life.

Harry grew up in New London, Connecticut, in a family of professional actors and models. His mother, a professional model, got him involved in the business at age five, appearing in commercials.

He enjoys traveling to tropical destinations, especially Hawaii, Bermuda, and the Caribbean. His favorite pastimes are dancing and collecting vintage vinyl records. Harry resides in New London's shoreline community.

Email: scriptproducerHLT@gmail.com
Facebook: @FindingPeacebytheSea
www.facebook.com/ACTORHLT
Twitter: @Thomas_Actor
Instagram: actor_ht
Vimeo: Harry Thomas Actor-Producer

www.ingramcontent.com/pod-product-compliance
Ingram Content Group UK Ltd.
Pitfield, Milton Keynes, MK11 3LW, UK
UKHW062302290726
14090UKWH00017B/837

9 781665 302920